Courtney's Healing Journey
Candida Overgrowth, Vaccine Injury, Heavy Metals
Poisoning, and Her Path to Victory
by Kim Seymour LVN and Courtney Seymour

Copyright 2020 by Kim Seymour LVN and Courtney
Seymour

Hope Kelley Book Publishing
HopeKelleyBookPublishing.com
publish@HopeKelley.com
800.806.6240

Printed in the United States of America

The material and nutritional education offered in *Courtney's
Healing Journey* are for informative purposes only. Neither
the publisher nor the authors shall be liable or legally
responsible for any loss or damage allegedly arising from the
use of any information or suggestions contained in this book.
This publication is intended to provide helpful information on
a healthy lifestyle by means of cleansing and restorative
methods. This information is not intended to diagnose nor
treat any disease.

Courtney's Healing Journey

Candida Overgrowth, Vaccine Injury, Heavy Metals Poisoning, and Her Path to Victory

by

Kim Seymour LVN

and

Courtney Seymour

Dedications

"I dedicate this book to those who are vaccine injured, because that is where I used to be and that is where my heart is. I would love to connect with those who are vaccine injured and tell you not to give up. I know it is hard but do not give up! You must keep fighting. God is there with you and I would love to be there for you, too. There were many times I wanted to give up, but God helped me to push through and He can help you to push through, too! I want to see people heal like I have! I would love to watch your healing journeys and celebrate your victories that God gives you! I remember being so scared that I was going to die, even after an Angel came to me at the foot of my bed and told me that I was not going to die. But it was hard to believe because of the way I felt. Then my mom prayed that God would heal me. Awhile after that, He told my mom He would heal me, and He did! God is a promise keeper. He also led us to the right supplements and the right people as you will read in this book. I will be praying for you. God promises to NEVER leave us NOR forsake us. He will help you get through this. God shows me that I am stronger than I think I am. Please do not give up. There is hope! You are not alone." ~~Courtney Seymour

"I dedicate this book to my brave daughter. Courtney, I admire you. Through your healing journey you have taught me about life. I have admired your determination to live. I have admired your dedication to your spiritual journey with God. I admire your zest for life and helping others who are on the same path that you have been on. You have been my light at the end of a long dark tunnel. I am so excited to be able to watch you from the front row and see how God is using you and will use you. Thank you for being open to Him and allowing Him to use you. I love you more than my words can say and more than I can ever express. I am so thankful He gave me the opportunity to be your mother." ~~Kim Seymour

"But as for you, ye thought evil against me; but God meant it unto good, to bring to pass, as it is this day, to save much people alive." Genesis 50:20 (KJV)

Foreword

Kim Seymour is an experienced and highly trained nurse, and my dear friend as well. Her daughter Courtney is the subject of this book. When Kim asked me to write the Foreword to *Courtney's Healing Journey* I was more than happy and honored. I immediately accepted. This story needed to be told and it is definitely one that every parent needs to hear.

Courtney's story is skillfully and thoroughly written. It illustrates that there is nothing more powerful than the love of a mother for her child. It was Kim's fierce dedication that eventually resulted in her daughter healing herself from the devastating injuries that were caused by vaccines.

Do not miss this compelling story.

~~ Jane Remington

Author of *Recaging The Beast*

Acknowledgements

There is no way Courtney and I can express our gratitude fully to all who have been the "wind beneath our wings." Thank you, many friends, who made it clear to us that there was a real need for this book about candida overgrowth, vaccine injury, and heavy metals poisoning.

With love and appreciation to Ernie and Ruby Saunders, Kim's parents and Courtney's grandparents. Thank you for your patience and support. Thank you for praying for Courtney and me as we wrote this book. Thank you for putting up with our achieving this goal, amid the kitchen table. It most definitely was not smooth sailing.

Thank you, Jane Remington, author of *Recaging the Beast*, for your support and most of all your loving friendship of several years. You will never know how much Courtney and I appreciate the time you took to read and edit our book. Sometimes we meet a rare individual who brings light into our lives. You, Jane Remington, are one of those rare individuals. You are an extraordinary teacher. You expanded our knowledge through *Recaging the Beast* and with our many phone calls of the importance of food and herbs and their healing effects in our bodies.

I want to take this opportunity to make a public apology to my daughter, Courtney. I am so sorry that I put you through this. I am sorry that I did not do my due diligence research, as your mother, and I was ignorant and gave into the chemicals and poisons that caused you to suffer. I praise God every day that He healed you and He showed me the right answers and individuals for your healing journey. I am blessed and honored that God chose me to be your mother. I love you.

Table of Contents

Chapter 1

I'm A Girl!

Courtney was born November of 1991. She was a healthy eight pounds, two and a half ounces and nineteen inches long. Her APGR was 7-9.

What does APGR mean?

Activity, Pulse, Grimace, Appearance, and Respiration.

According to https://www.babycenter.com/pregnancy/your-body/the-apgar-score_3074

"The Apgar score assesses your newborn's condition in the minutes after birth. The Apgar score is a simple numerical assessment that rates how a baby is doing at birth. The Apgar test helps the doctor quickly determine whether your newborn might need additional medical assistance. A score of 7 to 10 is considered normal for both the one-minute and five-minute Apgar tests."

In Courtney's baby book I have written that the president was George Bush.

I chose to breastfeed her. Her pediatrician told me to allow her to breastfeed for 10 minutes on each breast for each feeding and to feed her every two to three hours.

To my knowledge, she received all her newborn vaccines while in the hospital. Her skin was red. I asked the nurse why she was so red. I was told the redness was because of the trauma of her birth. However, she was only a three-hour labor and delivery. That did not settle well with me, but I took it and did not question it anymore.

As an infant, I took her to her pediatrician at least quarterly, if not more, because she was sick. Her pediatrician would frequently put her on an antibiotic. One day, I said to her pediatrician, "It seems like she is on an antibiotic frequently." His response was, "This is what I was taught in medical school, so this is what I do."

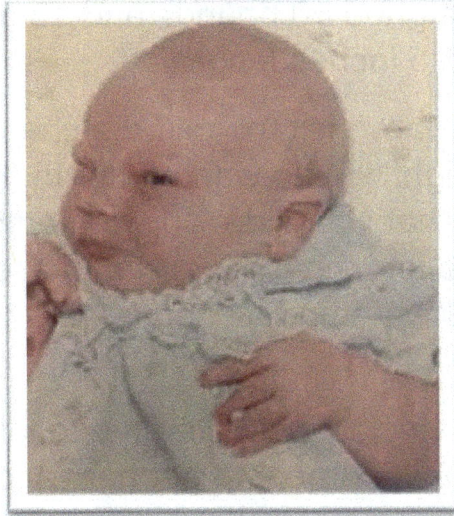

She hit some of her "milestones" a little late. According to her baby book, she started raising her head and rolling over at 2 months old, picking up and handling objects at 3 months old, sat up without support at 7 months old (about a month late), and crawling at 11 months old (about five months late). She started walking at a year and half and that was with much coaxing from her grandmama and me. Most babies start walking at around 9 months old. This may have been in part to her dad because he hated hearing her cry.

December 23, 1991, she was 1 month old. She weighed 9 pounds and 10 ounces and was 21 inches long. According to her vaccine record, January 21, 1992, she was 2 months old. She weighed 10 pounds and 13.5 ounces and was 21.5 inches long.

At her well baby visit, he told me she was not gaining weight like he wanted her to. He suggested that I consider supplementing with formula. He told me that we would see how much weight she had gained on her next well baby visit.

Her pediatrician instructed me to take her to the Health Department to get her vaccines. He gave me written instructions saying, "If she ran a fever to give her .3 of infant Tylenol. Give her .3 of infant Tylenol before and four hours after the vaccines are given. He also gave me written instructions indicating "POSSIBLE REACTIONS TO DPT". The paper stated, "There was a risk of reaction to DPT of 1:32 million and with polio the risk was 1:5 million. There is a great possibility that there will be a reaction to the injection. I should take her the ER if she has convulsions.

Possibilities are:

1) Fever of 100 to 103 or rarely 104 to 106.
2) Irritability and fussiness.
3) Painful swollen injection sites.
4) Crying Syndrome.
5) Convulsions.

Not: vomiting, spitting or diarrhea.

The reaction may last 24 to 36 hours. If there is fever and fussiness after the 2 doses of fever medication you may repeat it as long as the fever is present. Not any more often than every 3 to 4 hours. If the leg becomes red, swollen, and feverish, place a cold washcloth on it. Many times, a knot in the leg will result and may be present up to two weeks."

January 30, 1992, she received her 2-month vaccines. February 21, 1992, she was 3 months old. She weighed 11 pounds and 15 ounces and was 22 3/8 inches long. February 26, 1992, she was diagnosed with conjunctivitis (pink eye). She was given the DTP, Polio, and Hib CV #1.

March 23, 1992, she was 4 months old. She weighed 13 pounds 5 ¼ ounces and was 23 ¾ inches long. I was instructed by her pediatrician to take her to the Health Department for her vaccines and given the same written information as above. I was told to give her .4 infant Tylenol this time. March 26,1992, she received her 4-month vaccines. The DTP, Polio, and Hib #2. April 21, 1992, at 5 months old, she weighed 14 pounds and 7 ounces and was 25 inches long. We started her on baby food vegetables. May 21,1992, she received her 6-

month vaccines. The DTP and Hib #3. She weighed 14 pounds and 14.5 ounces and was 25 ½ inches in length. We started her on diluted juices, yogurt, cottage cheese, jello, and baby food meats.

June 27, 1992, she was diagnosed with an ear infection and tonsillitis. June 29, 1992, she was diagnosed with roseola because she broke out into a rash all over her body.

Was it really roseola? Or was it an allergic reaction that was misdiagnosed?

July 9, 1992, at 8 months old, she received the Polio vaccine. At 9 months old, she weighed 16 pounds and 3 ounces and was 26 ¾ inches in length. We started her on homogenized milk and Poly Vi Sol 1 cc/day. Poly Vi Sol is a pediatric liquid multivitamin with iron. We started experimenting with table foods and adult cereals (finger foods). He wanted her eating a complete egg twice a week.

December 11, 1992, she was 12 months old. She weighed 17 pounds and 10.5 ounces and was 28.5 inches long. December 14, 1992 she was diagnosed with rotavirus and hospitalized for dehydration due to profuse vomiting, diarrhea, and a high fever. They discharged her from the hospital December 18, 1992 after IV infusions to combat the dehydration.

I made the connection of the rotavirus with a recent well baby visit and spoke with her pediatrician's staff about it. After they looked at their records, they admitted that Courtney was seen right after a baby that was diagnosed with rotavirus and ended up in the hospital as well. They admitted that they were so busy that day that they did not sanitize the area. Instead, they just took the dirty paper off and replaced it with clean paper. The baby that was seen before Courtney did have a diarrhea diaper changed right before leaving.

In Courtney's baby book, at 12 months, I have documented that she was gritting her teeth at night during her sleep.

February 23, 1993 at 15 months old, she received DTP, Polio, MMR and Hib #4.

At her 4 months well baby visit, she was still not gaining enough weight, according to percentile.

What is percentile?

At a well-baby visit, the clinician will measure height, weight, and head circumference. That data will be plotted on the growth chart and compared to the "normal range" and to the child's own previous curve.

This is what you will typically be shown on a computer in the exam room.

I hesitantly agreed to supplement with formula. Of course, the bottle was easier for her and I started drying up.

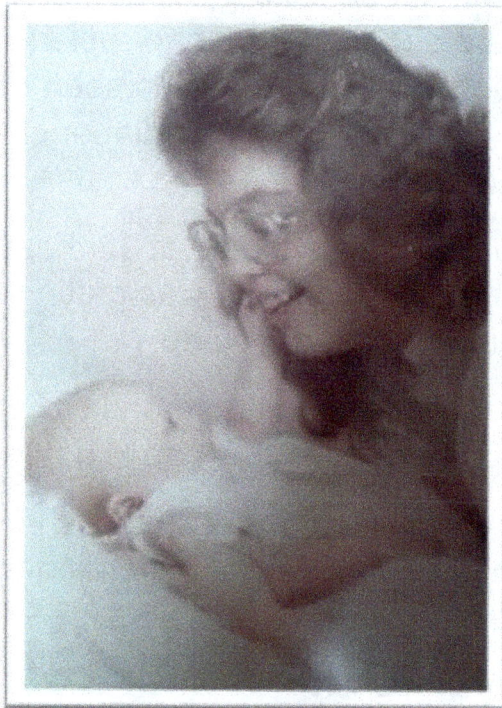

January 10, 1996, at 5 years old, she received DTP and OPV (oral polio).

I changed pediatricians because I was tired of spending my time in her pediatrician's office. October 1,1996, she contracted chicken pox.

This means she had immunity to the chicken pox! September 8, 1997, at the age of 6, she received the MMR.

In middle school she was classified as a "slow learner" and we placed her in some special education classes per her teachers' suggestions.

August 2, 2000, she received Hepatitis B #1. According to her records this was Merck's vaccine, and they gave it in her right thigh. October 5, 2000, she received Hepatitis B #2. According to records this was Merck's vaccine also, and it was given in her right thigh. January 16, 2001, she received an influenza vaccine and the Hepatitis B #3. According to records the influenza was Wyeth's vaccine given in her left arm and Hepatitis B was Merck's vaccine given in her right arm.

September 29, 2003, Courtney's school did a spine check on her and recommended that I take her to a special doctor for possible scoliosis. She had been complaining of her lower back hurting anyway. I took her to her pediatrician first and he recommended a specialist. The specialist diagnosed her with a moderate levorotoscoliosis of the lumbar spine with a 26-degree angulation involving T12 through L4.

December 3, 2005, I took her to urgent care for what looked like a spider bite on her left lateral calf. It turned out to be MRSA.

What is MRSA?

Methicillin-resistant Staphylococcus aureus (MRSA) is caused by a type of staph bacteria that has become resistant to many of the antibiotics used to treat ordinary staph infections. What is called Community-associated MRSA (CA-MRSA), often begins as a painful skin boil. It is spread by skin-to-skin contact. Courtney was taking a PE class at the time and she was sleeping with me. At the time, I worked at our local hospital. However, she had also been on a lot of antibiotics throughout her lifetime indicating antibiotic resistance.

What is antibiotic resistance?

The result of decades of often unnecessary antibiotic use. For years, antibiotics have been prescribed for colds, flu and other viral infections that do not respond to these drugs. Even when antibiotics are used appropriately, they contribute to the rise of drug-resistant bacteria because they do not destroy every germ they target. Bacteria live on a growing fast track, so germs that survive treatment with one antibiotic soon learn to resist others.

You can learn more about antibiotic resistance in our blog post at https://compassionwithkim.com/?p=969.

January 3, 2006, she received a DTP vaccine.

In October of 2006, I filed for divorce from her dad along with a protective order for our safety. It became final the summer of 2007. I had started dating a gentleman in the fall of 2007 and the doctor was blaming her stomach pain on stress caused by the divorce and her dad and I moving on with our lives with other people. We accepted that reason and we did our best to get on with our lives.

In 2007, she started having breathing difficulty during Physical Education (PE) class and was diagnosed with exercise induced asthma by her new pediatrician and put on two different inhalers. She was put on ProAir HFA CFC free 90 mcg/inh as needed and Symbicort 80 mcg-4.5 mcg/inh twice a day. Her pediatrician said, "We are not going to make a big deal out of this. All she needs is the inhalers." One inhaler was emergent (as needed), and the other inhaler was daily.

In high school she started to have stomach pain and on May 9, 2008 an esophagogastroduodenoscopy (EGD) was performed by a very well-known GI specialist for persistent epigastric pain with nausea and diarrhea. According to her medical records, Maalox, and proton pump inhibitors (PPI) were not taking care of her stomach pain. Her records indicated that she had been complaining of upper abdominal pain for four months! Her GI specialist told us the results were negative. He started her on a trial of anticholinergics. Courtney was 16 years old at the time.

What are anticholinergics?

Anticholinergics are drugs that block the action of acetylcholine. Acetylcholine is a neurotransmitter, or a chemical messenger. It transfers signals between certain cells to affect how your body functions.

Anticholinergics can treat a variety of conditions, including:

- Urinary incontinence
- Overactive bladder (OAB)
- Chronic obstructive pulmonary disorder (COPD)
- certain types of poisoning

They also help block involuntary muscle movements associated with certain diseases. Sometimes, they are used before surgery to help maintain body functions while a person is treated with anesthesia.

When we had exhausted all means with this well-known GI specialist, he referred Courtney to a Specialty Pediatric Gastroenterology in Lubbock, Texas. He found all testing to be negative as well.

December 21, 2009, Courtney was 18 years old and she received the Gardasil (HPV) vaccine #1, meningitis and Tdap. According to her records, the Gardasil was given in her right arm and the meningitis (Menactra) and Tdap were given in her left arm. She weighed 104 pounds. February 24, 2010, she received the Gardasil (HPV) vaccine #2. According to records it was given in her left arm.

Praise God, she graduated from high school on May 29, 2010!

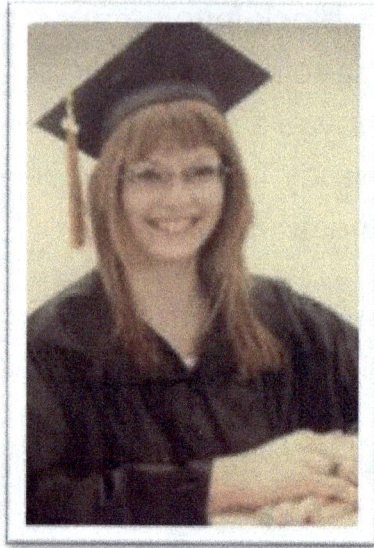

September 21, 2010, her pediatrician ordered a urine culture and some blood work. The urine culture resulted >100,000 CFU/ml group D enterococcus (infection). The Epstein-Barr virus (EBV) panel indicated VCA-IgG >750.0 (positive), VCA-IgM <10.0 (negative), early AG <5.0 (negative) and EBNA >600.0 (positive).

According to https://healthmysteriessolved.com/how-interpret-ebv-lab-results/ Courtney's results indicates past infection.

Why was I not told about this?

September 22, 2010, gran % is high at 78, lymph % low at 17 and lymph # low at 0.9.

These labs indicate that she had both a bacterial and viral infection.

September 29, 2010, she had a pelvic sonogram done per her pediatrician. We were told that it was negative. However, while writing this book and going through her medical records, we found that she had a right ovarian cyst that measured 14x7x10 mm. Apparently not big enough for them to do anything about.

At this point, I made the decision that since she was 18 years old, it was time to find a primary care physician (PCP) for her.

August 18, 2011, she saw her new primary care physician (PCP). Her blood work showed her WBC was low at 4.2. A low WBC is called leukopenia. A low number can be triggered by:

- HIV
- Autoimmune disorders
- bone marrow disorders or damage
- lymphoma
- severe infections
- liver and spleen diseases
- lupus

- radiation therapy
- some medications, such as antibiotics

Why was I not told about this?

They also did a urine culture which was positive for group B beta and she was treated with Keflex (antibiotic).

August 22, 2011, her urine culture from PCP indicates group B strep. Another dose of Keflex 500 mg three times a day for five days.

September 2, 2011, at her PCP, again. She did a urine culture and it indicated group B strep. She was started on yet another antibiotic.

September 6, 2011, another urine culture done and another group B strep diagnosis. And, yes, another antibiotic.

September 21, 2011, her PCP did a follow up urine culture via strait cath and it was negative! She still recommended for Courtney to see a urologist.

October 11, 2011, I took Courtney to a cardiologist. However, I have no record of what happened, only a receipt.

November 8, 2011, at the age of 19, she saw a urologist for recurrent bladder infections, urinary urgency and incomplete bladder emptying. Her weight at the time was 102 pounds. She has had three bladder infections in the last six months according to her PCP. They had all been treated with antibiotics. She had been getting up at least once during the night to urinate.

The urologist asked her if she could give a urine sample. After drinking some water, she was able to provide the sample, but she complained of not feeling empty. He decided to strait cath her and 220 ml's of residual urine came out!

December 15, 2011, I took Courtney to a pulmonologist. However, I do not have any record of what happened, only a receipt.

December 19, 2011, she did a urinalysis that showed "budding yeast". (While writing this book and looking through her medical records, I found where it stated that her urinalysis showed "budding yeast".)

Why was I not told about this?

This is an indication of candida overgrowth.

He said he could not find anything "wrong" and he ordered her to decrease her fluid intake. He referred her to an endocrinologist.

I decided against the endocrinologist. Based on my knowledge, at the time, I felt like it was a dead-end road.

She got married in November 2013. She was married without my blessing and I was not invited to her wedding. Her husband did not like me.

Chapter 2

Hitting Rock Bottom

Late 2014, over the period of approximately three months she frequently texted me informing me that she was losing weight and needing to go to the hospital via ambulance often. One day she texted me informing me that she was down to 81 pounds! Wow! She is five feet four inches tall! This was not good!

As her mother, and a western medicine nurse, I knew that it was time to take action, whether she and her husband approved or not.

I told her to eat sugar loaded and high fat foods in order to gain weight. I was oblivious to the facts about the TRUTH about nutrition, at the time. As a western medicine nurse, I was required to take one semester of nutrition. However, the course was not taken seriously, by the whole class. It was part of our basics and we called it a "goof off" class. It was a "step on the ladder to success". I suggested foods like ice cream, hamburgers, peanut butter and I even told her how to make her own milk shakes with the thought of 'anything to just get her to gain weight'!

I texted her back asking if she would be able to go out to eat with me, my treat. She said yes!

When I arrived to pick her up from her house, she came out and I saw that she was skin and bones. I remember thinking to myself, how on earth is she even walking? She was very pale, and a bit stooped over like she was having a hard time walking.

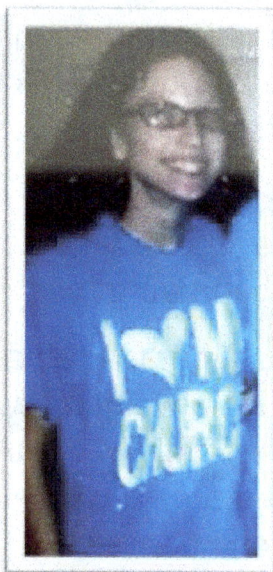

During our meal she began to open up to me informing me about what was going on with her health and her marriage. Her husband had to work that night, so I asked her if she would want to stay the night with me. She accepted my invitation!

Long story short, she ended up moving in with me and going through a divorce.

She was twenty-three years old and I could see that her health had been rapidly declining. She was experiencing severe chest pain and abdominal pain daily and multiple times a day.

I found out that before she moved in with me, she had applied for health care at a local health care clinic. I knew she needed to be seen by a doctor to get blood work done, so that I would be able to get some baseline health information. I needed to know what she was going through and what I was dealing with. She informed me that she was waiting for acceptance to this local health care clinic. I called the clinic and informed them of her condition and asked them if the acceptance process could be sped up. They informed me it could, so I took her to their urgent care in January of 2015.

At the urgent care, they took her vital signs, assessed her, and drew her blood for lab work. Her blood pressure was low, pulse was a little high, and her lab work indicated that her kidneys were shutting down. Her potassium level was low (hypokalemia), and it was affecting her heart. The Nurse Practitioner (NP) said she was not sick enough for hospital admission, but asked Courtney if she was afraid to go to sleep at night for fear that she would not wake up the next morning?

What?!

Courtney said "yes" and began a hard, blubbering cry.

I looked the NP in her eyes, and I said to her, "You have my full attention. What do we need to do?" She prescribed a bunch of medications, prayed with us, and sent us home informing me to, "Keep a very close eye on her."

Every night when we went to bed, I would tell myself, do not be surprised if you wake up and she has died during the night.

When she moved in, she was sleeping on the couch in my living room. She would frequently wake up during the night gasping for air and hollering at me because she was scared and having a hard time catching her breath. We made the decision to move her to the recliner in the living room because of her symptoms of GERD and sleep apnea. She asked me to start sleeping in the living room with her. I began sleeping on the couch.

On February 9, 2015, she had to go the ER for chest pain and dizziness. They diagnosed her with dehydration and anxiety. Her blood pressure was low, and they gave her IV fluids. They also checked her blood glucose and did an H. pylori antibody. All labs were negative. They told her to keep taking her vitamins.

What is an H. pylori antibody?

According to https://www.healthline.com/health/helicobacter-pylori

"H. pylori is a common type of bacteria that grows in the digestive tract and has a tendency to attack the stomach lining. H. pylori infections are usually harmless, but they are responsible for most ulcers in the stomach and small intestine.

The "H" in the name is short for Helicobacter. "Helico" means spiral, which indicates that the bacteria are spiral shaped."

February 16, 2015, she had to go the ER for chest pain. They did blood work, a drug screening, urinalysis, EKG and chest x-rays. They sent her home with Naproxen (anti-inflammatory), promethazine (nausea/vomiting) and Tramadol (pain). No cardiology orders were placed.

In a one-week period, I took Courtney to the ER five times for chest pain with abdominal pain. The ER would do the usual cardiac protocol work-up and everything came out negative, all five times. The last time, she was even accused of doing drugs and labeled a "drug seeker". We were told by the ER nurse that it was "time to accept that our lives would just be this way".

What? Why?!

As I was pushing her out the ER door in a wheelchair, with her bent over in abdominal pain and crying, I was crying too. I could not believe they were going to send her home in this much pain! How was I going to get her pain under control by myself at home?

I noticed as I was pushing her out to our car that the two ER staff members that sit at the front desk were laughing at us and saying that Courtney was faking it. As a nurse I thought, how could they be so mean?

As an inquisitive nurse, I wanted to know WHY our lives were suddenly being turned upside down. WHY was my child suddenly having chest pain and abdominal pain at only twenty-three years of age?

Chapter 3

The Phone Call

Late February 2015, Courtney was set up with a PCP through the local health care clinic. Her stomach was still hurting multiple times a day, so they did an x-ray. The x-ray showed "significant gastroesophageal reflux disease (GERD) to the level of the proximal esophagus, and a limited coating of the stomach and esophagus."

A dysphagiagram or swallow evaluation was ordered because she was having a hard time swallowing food and pills.

At this time, she was given a GI specialist and, after assessing Courtney, he decided not to do a swallow evaluation and instead he ordered a gastric emptying study. The gastric emptying study findings were "gastric emptying is prolonged".

I felt like she needed an esophagogastroduodenoscopy (EGD) and the GI specialist agreed to do an EGD. However, before the EGD, he wanted to do a CT scan.

April 3, 2015, a CT scan of her abdomen was performed that showed "a moderate to large pericardial effusion has increased in size since the prior CT. The effusion extends along the base of the heart. There may be thickening of the gastroesophageal junction. The presence of an esophagitis cannot be excluded from this. Dr. has been notified".

Her GI specialist called me at home and informed me that the CT showed fluid on her heart! He told us to go to the ER and a cardiologist was already assigned to her and to ask for him and they were going to possibly admit her through the ER depending on what the cardiologist said. Therefore, we needed to prepare for a possible hospital stay.

I got off the phone and told Courtney. Courtney and I began crying and hugging each other. Could this be the relief she needs? We said a quick prayer together ("For where two or three have gathered together in My name, I am there in their midst." Matthew 18:20 (NAS)) and I started packing. While I was packing, I thought, increased in size since the prior CT? What CT?

When we arrived at the ER, we were told the fluid had been there for a while and it was being SECRETLY monitored! We were told they are not supposed to take fluid off the heart until it reaches a certain amount!

Do you remember Courtney and I leaving the ER and the two staff members sitting at the desk laughing and saying she was faking it? You should have seen the looks on their faces when we walked in and let them know we were there to meet this cardiologist! They recognized Courtney!

After arriving to the ER and meeting with the cardiologist, thankfully a very well-known cardiologist, I informed him that she was diagnosed with influenza B about two weeks prior. Courtney did receive a flu shot before she contracted the flu.

According to her hospital records, at 2 PM her blood pressure (BP) was 121/77, heart rate (HR) 126, respiratory rate (RR) 20 and oxygen saturation (O2 sat) 99% on room air (RA). They asked Courtney what her weight and height were. She said 5 feet 3 inches and 83 pounds. Her body mass index (BMI) was calculated at 14.25. If she were at her ideal weight of 120 pounds, her BMI would be about 22. They asked her what is the most she had ever weighed. She said 105 pounds. I later corrected her and told her the most she had ever weighed had been 110 pounds. However, 105 pounds was charted. Therefore, a 22-pound unintended weight loss was documented.

A nursing plan of care (POC) of chest pain was initiated. At 2:30 she started complaining of chest pain and rated it at a 7. A stat EKG, chest x-ray and an echocardiogram (echo) were ordered. They, of course, did the usual cardiac workup.

Her diagnosis was a pericarditis with a large pericardial effusion without tamponade physiology.

A pericarditis is the swelling and irritation of the thin saclike membrane surrounding the heart. When the pericardium becomes injured or affected by infection, fluid can build up between its delicate layers. This condition is called pericardial effusion.

Cardiac tamponade is where the fluid in the sac around the heart builds up, resulting in compression of the heart. A collection of three medical signs associated with cardiac tamponade, are low blood pressure, distended neck veins, and shortness of breath. All signs that Courtney was experiencing, except for the distended neck veins. Therefore, tamponade was dismissed.

Her HR was 126. I asked her cardiologist, "How did the fluid get on her heart?" He said he did not know. I asked him, "Did the flu shot cause the fluid to get on her heart?" He said he did not know.

Courtney told her nurse that the GERD was worse after meals and her chest pain would last all day and sometimes be continuous for days. At this point her HR was 141. Their records from the health care clinic indicated that she had been having chest pain, shortness of breath and palpitations for three months! She also had an unintended ten-pound weight loss in the last three months with occasional constipation.

She had the prior CT done early January that we were told was negative!

Her doctor said the CT performed on this day showed GERD as well as worsening of the pericardial effusion compared to early January when she had a small pericardial effusion.

At 2:20 her sodium was high at 141, potassium was low at 3.3, carbon dioxide (CO_2) was low at 20.0 and her platelet (plt) clumps was 1+.

Platelet clumps are abnormal platelet clumping that can damage organs.

At 3:00 she was experiencing heartburn and rated her chest pain at a 4. At 4:30 an echocardiogram (echo) was performed. It showed left ventricular ejection fraction of 60% to 65%. She had a "moderate pericardial effusion with no clear evidence of tamponade physiology. Effusion is approximately 2 cm and adjacent to right-sided chambers."

In the charting, her cardiologist noted that he suspected that it was secondary to recent influenza.

He did not want to drain the fluid off her heart, instead he started her on Allopurinol as an off-label use, 1.2 mgs daily.

Off-label use is the use of pharmaceutical drugs for an unapproved indication or in an unapproved age group, dosage, or route of administration. As a western medicine nurse, this did not alarm me because we practiced this at a local hospital where I used to work. However, I found out years later, that off-label use means that the manufacturer of the medicine had not applied for a license for it to be used to treat the condition. In other words, the medicine has not undergone clinical trials to see if it is effective and safe in treating her condition. If I had known this at the time, I would have never allowed this.

He informed me he wanted to try it for four days and see if it would take the fluid off her heart. He looked at her labs and saw that she was in metabolic acidosis. He suspected renal (kidney) tubular acidosis from impaired renal bicarbonate resorption. In other words, she is acidic, and it is causing her kidneys to shut down. He ordered more labs to evaluate her kidney function. He also noticed that her hands were red and suspected Raynaud's, therefore he ordered labs to check for that as well.

Metabolic acidosis occurs when the body produces too much acid. It can also occur when the kidneys are not removing enough acid from the body. Renal tubular acidosis (RTA) is a disease that occurs when the kidneys fail to excrete acids into the urine, which causes a person's blood to remain too acidic.

Raynaud's disease, or RD, is an autoimmune condition that causes the ends of the toes and fingers to feel cold, numb and tingly. Blood vessels in the hands and feet appear to overreact to cold temperatures and/or stress, which constricts blood flow to the affected tissue. The skin can change colors, from white to blue to red, and is more likely to affect those who live in colder climates.

At 5:30 they ordered to encourage intake on clear liquid diet and advance her to a regular diet as tolerated and to obtain her weight every three days. At 7:30 they ordered a stat ANA, antibody, lupus, Sjogren's, random urine sodium, random urine potassium, random urine chloride and D dimer ultrasensitive.

At 8 PM they decided to admit her to the hospital. Finally! She was admitted with a heart monitor. The doctor wrote two standing orders: 1) Order a STAT potassium level 2 hours after total regimen of potassium is administered and notify provider if below 2.5 mEq/L for the next 72 hours. 2) Order a magnesium level if potassium level remains below 3.6 mEq/L after first potassium replacement series and notify provider with result for the next 72 hours.

Praise God, she was negative for lupus and Sjogren's!

At 9:15 they did another EKG, and her HR was 84. Courtney had been dealing with some nasal congestion and they thought it might have been adding to the situation. The doctor ordered some sodium chloride nasal spray. At 9:20 she was given Tylenol 2 tabs/650 mgs, potassium chloride 20 mEq and Colchicine 2 tabs at 1.2 mg/tab. At 9:30 her BP is 101/72.

At 10:00 she was experiencing fatigue, palpitations, drowsiness, nausea, weakness and all extremities were cool. At 10:15 she was given Mylanta (Aluminum hydroxide/Magnesium hydroxide/simethicone) 5 ml oral suspension. At 10:30 her nurse charted that her left and right dorsalis pedis (top of feet) pulses are thready (weak) and she was experiencing heartburn. Her nurse charted that she received her flu vaccine prior to admission during the current flu season.

At 10:51 a nursing POC of at risk for falls and bowel dysfunction was initiated. At 11:30 she complained of nasal congestion and was given a saline nasal spray.

While writing this book I noticed that the nurse had charted that she had no cough, yet she was having bloody sputum. How does that happen? You cannot have bloody sputum without a cough. Besides, she was not having bloody sputum!

The medications that she was on at home, prior to admission, are as follows:

Multivitamin 1 tab daily

Naproxen 375 mg tab twice daily as needed for pain.

MiraLAX (laxative) 17 gm daily

Phenergan 25 mg tab every four hours as needed for nausea/vomiting.

Tramadol 50 mg tab every four hours as needed for pain.

While writing this book, I discovered in her medical records that at midnight her urine chloride was low at <52 (reference range 168-301) indicating congestive heart failure (CHF), vomiting or diarrhea. Her urine potassium level was low at 5.5 (reference range 27.0-129.0) indicating acidity, digestive issue and absorption problems. And her urine sodium level was low at 38 (reference range 53-236) indicating kidney problems.

Chapter 4

Her Hospital Admission

She was admitted into the hospital with a telemetry unit (records what the heart is doing) and severe, chronic gastroesophageal reflux disease (GERD) with severe shortness of breath on exertion, palpitations, chest pressure and multiple episodes of nausea and vomiting.

While writing this book, I discovered in her medical records that the doctor had suggest critical care placement. Because of all of this, she was, of course, experiencing depression and anxiety. This is the kind of stuff eighty-year-old elderly people deal with! Courtney was in her early 20's! She should have been out having fun with her friends! Why was she experiencing all this? The depression was because this had been going on for so long, at least three months, according to records. The anxiety was because nobody understood why this was happening to her. She was scared! And so was I.

Upon admission Allopurinol (usually used for gout but Courtney was using it off-label), Protonix (proton pump inhibitor to decrease acid in the stomach) and Zoloft 25 mg (antianxiety) were ordered to be given daily. Her as needed (PRN) orders were Tylenol 650 mg, Mylicon (gas) 80 mg as needed, simethicone (antacid) 30 ml as needed, BuSpar 5 mg twice a day as needed (anxiety), Toradol (pain), Zofran (nausea), magnesium sulfate protocol IV, potassium chloride protocol IV and/or 20 meq oral and simethicone for gas relief as well. The doctor ordered a dietitian referral. Her intake had been recorded at 150 ml's and her output 250 ml's.

April 4 at 00:30 she complained of chest pain and was given Tylenol 2 tabs (650 mg) and Zofran 4 mg via IV push for nausea. Her BP was 87/67, RR 15, HR 72, and O2 sat 98% on room air. The cardiac chest pain protocol was ordered consisting of a stat troponin every six hours for three times, a D-dimer, magnesium level, and potassium level.

The D-dimer result was <150. The doctor charted, "Patient states chest pain/pressure 9/10 radiating to left neck and arm accompanied by nausea and palpitations. EKG viewed, heart sounds normal, pulses normal. Will continue to evaluate for worsening symptoms of pericardial effusion."

Throughout this chapter, I am going to include some vital sign readings. Please pay close attention to them, as they are significant. Keep in mind, you may want to write these down or highlight them for reference, "average" vital signs are blood pressure (BP) 120/80, heart rate (HR) 60-100, respiratory rate (RR) 12-20, and oxygen saturation (O2 sat) 90-100%.

At 1:15 AM the medication was effective. A nursing POC for acute pain was initiated. At 2:00 her BP was 89/67, HR 84, RR 16, and O2 sat 100% on RA. At 3:00 her BP was 85/56, HR 79, RR 17 and O2 sat 100% on RA. At 4:23 her BP was 87/67, HR 83, and O2 sat 99% on RA.

Another nursing POC that was initiated was risk for decreased cardiac tissue perfusion. The doctor ordered to chart her mean arterial pressure.

What is mean arterial pressure?

Blood pressure monitors give you a systolic and diastolic blood pressure reading. Many monitors also include a small number in parentheses underneath or beside your standard blood pressure reading. This number in parentheses is the mean arterial pressure (MAP).

MAP is a calculation that doctors use to check whether there is enough blood flow, resistance, and pressure to supply blood to all your major organs.

"Resistance" refers to the way the width of a blood vessel impacts blood flow. For example, it is harder for blood to flow through a narrow artery. As resistance in your arteries increases, blood pressure also increases while the flow of blood decreases.

You can also think of MAP as the average pressure in your arteries throughout one cardiac cycle, which includes the series of events that happen every time your heart beats.

What is an "average" MAP?

In general, most people need a MAP of at least 60 mmHg (millimeters of mercury) or greater to ensure enough blood flow to vital organs, such as the heart, brain, and kidneys. Doctors usually consider anything between 70 and 100 mmHg to be "normal".

A MAP in this range indicates that there is enough consistent pressure in your arteries to deliver blood throughout your body.

What is a high MAP?

A high MAP is anything over 100 mmHg, which indicates that there is a lot of pressure in the arteries. This can eventually lead to blood clots or damage to the heart muscle.

Many things that cause high blood pressure can also cause a high MAP, including:

- Heart attack
- Kidney failure
- Heart failure

Courtney's problem at this point was kidney failure.

What is low MAP?

Anything under 60 mmHg is usually considered a low MAP. It indicates that your blood may not be reaching your major organs.

Without blood and nutrients, the tissue of these organs begins to die, leading to organ damage.

Doctors usually consider a low MAP to be a possible sign of:

- sepsis
- stroke
- internal bleeding

Courtney's potential problem was sepsis.

How is an unusual MAP treated?

An unusual MAP is usually a sign of an underlying condition or problem in the body, so treatment depends on the cause.

For a low MAP, treatment focuses on safely raising blood pressure quickly to avoid organ damage. This is usually done with:

- intravenous (IV) fluids or blood transfusions to increase blood flow
- medications called "vasopressors" that tighten blood vessels, which can increase

blood pressure and make the heartbeat faster or pump harder

Treating a high MAP also requires quick action, in this case, to reduce overall blood pressure. This can be done with oral or intravenous (IV) nitroglycerin (Nitrostat). This medication helps to relax and widen blood vessels, making it easier for blood to reach the heart.

Once blood pressure is under control, the doctor can begin treating the underlying cause. This might involve:

- breaking up a stroke-causing blood clot

- inserting a stent into a coronary artery to keep it open

The bottom line

MAP is an important measurement that accounts for flow, resistance, and pressure within your arteries. It allows doctors to evaluate how well blood flows through your body and whether it is reaching all your major organs.

At 5:00 AM her mean arterial pressure (MAP) was 61, BP 79/55, HR 81 and O2 sat 99% on RA. At 6:00 her MAP was 58 and BP 82/51.

Her sodium was higher at 144, potassium was better at 3.4, chloride was high at 116.0, calcium osmolality was high at 287 and anion gap was low at 6 (a low anion gap is rare). At 7 she was given Zofran 4 mg via IV push for nausea. At 7:30 her doctor came in to examine her and she said that she was hurting all over. She was given Tylenol 2 tabs (650 mg).

She reported to the doctor that she had chest pain during the night. He said he was going to order additional labs including a magnesium level protocol. He also ordered Zofran 2 mg/ml IV every 4 hours as needed for nausea/vomiting, Toradol 30 mg IV every 8 hours for pain, a 250 ml NS bolus to run over 30 minutes (to raise her blood pressure), a daily multivitamin, Naproxen 375 mgs twice daily as needed for pain and a TB test.

He said her rheumatoid factor (RF) was negative!

Rheumatoid factors are proteins produced by your immune system that can attack healthy tissue in your body. High levels of rheumatoid factor in the blood are most often associated with autoimmune diseases.

At 8:00 AM her MAP was 72 and BP 89/66. At 8:30 telemetry recorded her HR at 99. The Tylenol she took was effective! At 8:45 her nurse gave her an NS bolus 250 ml via IV and Mylanta (Al hydroxide/Mg hydroxide/simethicone) 5 ml oral suspension. At 9:00 her nurse charted that her left and right dorsalis pedis pulses were thready, she was having palpitations and all four extremities were cool. She was also experiencing heartburn and fatigue.

At 9:45 Tramadol 50 mgs oral every 4 hours was ordered for pain. At 10:00 her doctor ordered a TSH and an HIV test. The HIV test was negative, and the TB test was positive. Her nurse gave her a multivitamin 1 tab, sodium chloride nasal spray 2 sprays and Zoloft (antianxiety) 25 mg tab. Her MAP was 74, BP 99/67, HR 93, RR 25 and O2 sat 100% on RA.

At 10:10 her nurse charted that her left and right dorsalis pedis pulses were thready. She was also experiencing heartburn and weakness. She was given Colchicine 1 tab (0.6 mg).

At 12:45 PM her nurse gave her Zofran 4 mg via IV push for nausea. At 1:12 the Zofran was effective! Her BP was 92/63, HR 112, RR 21, and O2 sat 99% on RA. At 2:00 she was given Mylanta (Al hydroxide/Mg hydroxide/simethicone) 30 ml oral suspension for heartburn. At 3:00 PM she was given Tramadol 50 mg tab for a pain level of 6.

At 5:00 her MAP was 67, BP 95/57, HR 82, RR 20 and O2 sat 94% on RA. At 5:53 the Tramadol was effective! At 6:10 she was given Zofran 4 mg IV push. At 6:30 the Zofran was not effective. At 7:30 she was complaining of nausea and she was weak. Her nurse charted that Courtney was experiencing a lack of appetite. She was given Mylanta (Al hydroxide/Mg hydroxide/simethicone) 5 ml oral suspension for heartburn and Tramadol 50 mg tab for a pain level of 7.

At 8:30 Tramadol had brought her pain level down to a 2 and she was given sodium chloride nasal spray, 2 sprays. At 9:15 she was given Zofran 4 mg via IV push. At 9:45 she was given Toradol 1 ml IV push for a pain level of 5. At 10:15 the Toradol had brought her pain level down to a 3 and the Zofran was effective! At 11:00 the doctor ordered Protonix 40 mg via IV daily and Tums 500 mg oral every eight hours as needed for indigestion. At 11:10 she was given Mylanta 30 ml oral suspension, Protonix 40 mg IV push and Tramadol 50 mg tab for a pain level of 5. Her intake was recorded as 1,475 ml's and her output 1,425 ml's.

April 5, at 3:30 she was given Mylanta 30 ml oral suspension for heartburn. At 4:05 she was given Zofran 4 mg IV push for nausea. At 4:30 the Zofran was effective, and she was given a 500 ml NS bolus because her blood pressure was 84/51.

Her glucose was high at 118, sodium was high but better at 141, chloride was high but better at 113, CO_2 was low but better at 21, anion gap was low but better at 7, BUN/Creatine Ratio (kidney lab) was high at 21.25. At 5:00, her MAP was 68 and blood pressure 91/52. Her nurse notified her doctor, and a 500 ml bolus of Normal Saline (NS) was ordered to run via IV for 60 minutes.

It was charted that Courtney was having no complaints of shortness of breath or chest pain; however, she did say that her "GERD is starting to act up again." The doctor ordered a dietitian referral because she had been complaining of nausea for more than 72 hours.

At 7:30 she was complaining of nausea, cramping and heartburn. She was also very drowsy. Her nurse charted nutrition risk factor due to nausea or vomiting greater than 72 hours. At 8:50, she was given Protonix 40 mg

IV push, a multivitamin 1 tab, sodium chloride nasal spray 2 sprays, Zofran 4 mg IV push, Zoloft 25 mg tab, MiraLAX 17 gm oral and Colchicine 0.6 mg tab. At 9:20, the Zofran was effective!

At 10:00, the doctor came in and Courtney reported that she was fatigued and having decreased activity due to midsternal chest pain. She was also experiencing shortness of breath when walking to the bathroom. She was having pain with urination. Her potassium level was still low. He ordered a chest x-ray for her shortness of breath and added MiraLAX 17 gm oral daily for constipation, indomethacin (NSAID) 50 mg oral twice daily, Protonix 40 mg oral daily, Carafate 1 gm oral 4 times daily for GERD, multivitamin daily and Phenergan PRN.

At 10:05 she was given Naproxen 375 mg tab for a pain level of 6. At 11:05 the Naproxen had brought her pain level down to a 2.

At noon, her cardiologist came in and she was still having chest pain. Still without the classic features of cardiac tamponade. However, she was experiencing hypotension (low blood pressure) and shortness of breath. Her blood pressure was 98/62. He said the pericarditis was probably post flu but inflammatory was possible. He said she was still in metabolic acidosis with possible renal tubular acidosis.

At 1:10 PM she was given Phenergan 25 mg tab and Carafate (coats the stomach) 1 gm tab. At 1:45 she was given indomethacin (anti-inflammatory) 50 mg/2 caps. At 2:10 the Phenergan was effective! At 2:50 she was given Toradol 1ml via IV push for a pain level of 8. At 3:20 the Toradol reduced her pain level to a 4.

At 4:20 she had a chest x-ray. At 7:05 her nurse gave her Carafate 1 gm/tab. At 8:15 she was complaining of nausea, cramping and heartburn. At 8:20 her nurse gave her Zofran 4 mg IV push and Tylenol 650 mg/2 tabs for an epigastric pain level of 4. At 9:20 the Tylenol had brought her pain level down to a 2. At 8:50 the Zofran was working for her. At 10:35 she was given Toradol 1 ml IV push for a pain level of 5. At 11:10 the Toradol had lowered her pain level to a 1. Her intake was recorded at 600 ml's and output 500 ml's.

April 6, at midnight she had a bowel movement, and her stool was green probably because of food or medication. She was given sodium chloride nasal spray, Carafate 1 gm tab and Phenergan 25 mg tab. At 1:05 the Phenergan was working! At 3:55 she was given Zofran 4 mg IV push and Tylenol 650 mg/2 tabs. At 4:19 a nursing POC was initiated for at risk of pressure sore. At 4:25 the Zofran was working for her and the Tylenol had brought her pain level down to a 2.

She weighed 83.7 pounds! She had gained 7 ounces! Her BMI was 14.38. Her sodium was higher at 142, and chloride was high but better at 112, RBC was low at 3.95, anion gap was low but better at 8, BUN/Creatinine Ratio was even higher at 27.14, total protein (TP) was low at 5.8, Hemoglobin (Hgb) low at 11.7, Hematocrit (Hct) was low at 35 and alkaline phosphatase was low at 41.

A low Hgb and HCT will mean that there is insufficient oxygen circulating throughout the body. A low total protein level can occur for a variety of reasons that fall into the general categories of dilution, increased blood loss, decreased blood production and malnutrition. Low alkaline phosphatase (ALP) means her liver was compromised. Low levels of ALP indicate a great variety of problems: malnutrition, hypothyroidism, scurvy, deficiency of the essential mineral nutrients zinc and magnesium, anemia, and others.

At 5:00 AM the Tylenol had brought her pain level down to a 3. At 6:08 she was given Phenergan 25 mg tab and Toradol 1 ml IV push for a pain level of 3. At 6:38 the Toradol had brought her pain level down to a 2. At 7:10 the Phenergan was working for her. At 8:15 she was given Tylenol 650 mg/2 tabs and Zofran 4 mg IV push. At 8:45 she was given Zoloft 25 mg tab, Protonix 40 mg tab, Colchicine 0.6 mg tab, Mylanta 30 ml oral suspension (liquid), Carafate 1 gm tab and a multivitamin.

At 9:00 her doctor came in and she was complaining of chest pain that was radiating to her left shoulder. He informed me of her lab results. The rheumatoid arthritis (RA) and human immunodeficiency viruses (HIV) were negative! Her thyroid stimulating hormone (TSH) was "within normal limits". He increased the indomethacin dose and informed me her hypokalemia (low potassium) had been corrected.

At 9:15 AM her nurse charted that the Tylenol was effective with a pain level of a 6. What? How was that effective?

At 10:30 she was having chest pain with palpitations. Her HR was 76 with a regular rhythm and her pain was radiating down both arms. She was complaining of nausea and heartburn and her nurse charted that her arms and legs were restless. At 11:00 she was given

Phenergan 25 mg tab, sodium chloride nasal spray, and indomethacin 50 mg cap.

Just about the time I wanted to say, enough already, her cardiologist came in at 11:18 and she was still having chest pain. He had a recording of her episode from earlier that morning. He stated it was still without features of tamponade (hypotension, neck vein distension, and shortness of breath). The only symptom that was missing was the neck vein distension. I asked him if we could go ahead and do something different. Courtney had suffered enough. He informed me that he wanted to repeat the echo to see if there was a need for evacuation of pericardium.

At 11:40 the Phenergan was effective! She was 5 feet 4 inches tall and weighed 83 pounds.

Her nurse came in at 12:36 PM and Courtney was lying in bed with the head of the bed elevated and had a chest pain level of 8 with nausea. She was medicated with Zofran 4 mg IV push and Tylenol 650 mg/2 tabs. I was getting angry again that something more was not being done.

At 2:00 she was complaining of heartburn. At 2:40 she was given Carafate 1gm tab, Indocin 50 mg/2 caps, Mylicon 80 mg tab and Phenergan 25 mg tab. At 3:30 the usual cardiac protocol of troponin, CK and CK-MB were drawn, again, every 6-hour intervals for 3 times. At 3:40 the Phenergan and Zofran were effective, and the Tylenol had lowered her pain to a 4.

At 4:30 her CK was low at 28. Reference range is 38-234. A low level indicates low muscle mass or muscle atrophy and inflammation in autoimmune disorders.

At 6:10 she was given Tylenol 650 mg/2 tabs and Zofran 4 mg IV push. At 6:40 she was given Carafate 1 gm tab and the Zofran was charted as effective. At 7:15 the Tylenol was effective! At 8:15 she was complaining of nausea, cramping and heartburn. The nurse charted nutrition risk factors, nausea or vomiting greater than 72 hours.

At 9:38 PM she was given Phenergan 25 mg tab, Indocin 50 mg tab and sodium chloride nasal spray. At 10:40 the Phenergan was charted as effective and she was given Mylicon 80 mg tab. At 11:00 her CK was even lower at 25. Her input had been recorded as 2,400 ml's and output 2,100 ml's.

April 7, at midnight her MAP was 66 and BP 89/50. Her chloride was high but holding at 112, her WBC was low at 3.5, RBCs were lower at 3.89, Hgb was holding but Hct was lower at 34, anion gap lower yet at 6, BUN/Creatine Ratio higher yet at 23.33 and alkaline phosphatase lower yet at 39.0.

At 00:45 her BP went down to 89/50. Her doctor was notified, but he did not give any new orders. At 5:40 she was given Zofran 4 mg IV push and Tylenol 650 mg/2 tabs. At 5:50 she was given Carafate 1 gm tab. At 6:11 the Zofran was effective! At 6:30 the Zofran and Tylenol were charted as effective with a pain scale of 1.

At 7:09, her weight was 86.2 pounds! She had gained another 2.5 pounds! Her total gain now was 3.2 pounds! Her BMI was 14.8.

At 8:00, her doctor came in and she was complaining of heartburn, cramping and nausea. She was having chest pain radiating to her left shoulder with palpitations and she was rating it at a 3. The nurse charted that her pain was aggravated by movement. Courtney described her pain as aching, burning, heavy and radiating. Her doctor ordered the usual cardiac work up protocol labs. He informed me that the systemic lupus erythematosus (SLE) and scleroderma were negative! We are waiting on the repeated echo results. Her nurse gave her Protonix 40 mg tab, a multivitamin, and Colchicine 0.6 mg tab.

At 7:50 AM her CK was even lower at 20. At 8:10 she was given sodium chloride nasal spray and Zoloft 25 mg tab. At 9 her nurse charted sinus tachycardia (elevated heart rate) of 107 and PVCs.

PVC means premature ventricular contraction. I was so relieved that this was finally caught on paper because she had been experiencing palpitations for several months at home.

At 9:35 she was given Indocin 50 mg/2 caps. At 10:30 she was given Tylenol 650 mg/2 tabs. At 11:15 she was given Carafate 1 gm tab, Mylanta 30 ml oral suspension, and Zofran 4 mg IV push. At 11:45 the Zofran and Tylenol were charted as effective with a pain level of 3.

At 11:51 her cardiologist came in and she was still having pain and it was happening RANDOMLY. However, she was doing better. He informed me that her repeated echo had resulted showing left ventricular ejection fraction greater than 60%. It now shows moderate pericardial effusion, suggestive of tamponade physiology with presystolic collapse of mid to apical right ventricle with tamponade physiology. He finally decided he wanted to pursue a pericardial window. He said he had contacted a cardiac surgeon to do the surgery and she would be in to consult.

Finally!

At 1:15 PM she was given Phenergan 25 mg tab. At 2:00, Courtney was in bed with the head of the bed elevated and she was experiencing a pain level of 10. Her pain was in her chest radiating down both arms, up her neck, abdomen and down both legs. She described her pain as burning, pressure, pins and needles. Her pain started with walking to the bathroom. Her nurse medicated her with Tylenol 650 mg/2 tabs and notified her physician. She was tachycardic with a heart rate ranging between 92-120's. After her physician was notified, she was given a one-time dose of 2 mg morphine via IV. I began to wonder if she was going to have surgery a bit earlier than planned.

At 2:15 PM the Phenergan was charted as effective and she was given Mylicon 80 mg tab. At 2:53 she was rating her pain at a 10. At 3:00 she was given Mylanta 30 ml oral suspension and Morphine 2 mg IV push. At 4:00 the cardiac surgeon ordered ABO+Rh (blood type) and an antibody screen and then canceled them. Then she ordered them again. She also ordered an HCG Qual Urine (pregnancy test), pericardial window consent and NPO (nothing by mouth) at midnight.

It has been determined that her blood type is A+. At 4:30 the Morphine was effective with a pain level of 1. The Tylenol was charted as effective with a pain level of 4. What? The Tylenol did nothing for her pain! She had to have the Morphine to get her pain under control!

At 5:45 she was being given a tablet and she started choking on it. Her nurse called the doctor and asked to change the medication tablet to a liquid. He said it was fine.

At 6:50 she was having chest pain and rating it at an 8. They ordered her sucralfate 10 ml oral 4 times a day. At 7:00 PM her pregnancy test came back negative. We knew it would.

At 7:11 she got choked on another tablet. At 7:30 she was experiencing nausea and heartburn. She was given sodium chloride nasal spray and Carafate 10 ml. She was experiencing chest pain but only rates it at a 1. The nurse charted nutrition risk factors, nausea or vomiting greater than 72 hours.

At 8:05 she was given Indocin 50 mg/2 caps and the Tylenol was effective with a pain level of 1. At 8:50 she was given Tylenol 650 mg/2 tabs. At 9:00 she was given Zofran 4 mg IV push. At 9:30 the Zofran was effective! At 10:50 she was given Tylenol 650 mg/2 tabs for pain.

At 10:58 she was having chest pain and rating it at an 8. She described the pain as sharp and radiating down her left arm, upper back and neck. Her doctor was notified. At 11:10 the cardiac surgeon ordered 4 mg morphine IV for pain. At 11:22 the nurse charted a nursing POC of impaired gas exchange. At 11:56 the morphine brought her pain level down to a 2. The nurse made her NPO (nothing by mouth) in preparation for surgery. Her intake was recorded as 1,891.25 ml's and output 1,900 ml's.

Chapter 5

Prepping for Surgery

April 8, at midnight her MAP was 66, BP 88/55, respiratory rate (RR) 18 and O2 sat 97% on room air (RA). At 2:00 AM she was given morphine 4 mg IV push for a pain level of 8. Her RR was 20. At 2:30 the morphine was effective, and her pain was reduced to a 2.

Her potassium was low again at 3.4, chloride was higher again at 113, anion gap was even lower at 4, and BUN/creatine ratio was high but better at 26.67. At 4:00 AM, the nurse came in with a 40 meq dose of potassium chloride oral. I refused it and insisted on IV since she was NPO for surgery. At 5:00 the nurse came in with 40 meq potassium chloride with 250 ml NS IV to be given over 4 hours. At 5:05 she was given Zofran 4 mg IV push. At 8:00 her doctor diagnosed her as having pericardial effusion with tamponade and right ventricular collapse.

This day had finally come!

I gave her a chlorhexidine bath and the nurse helped with a complete linen change to get Courtney ready for surgery. Chlorhexidine is a disinfectant and antiseptic that is used for skin disinfection before surgery. Courtney was complaining of GERD, so her nurse gave her a one-time dose of Protonix 40 mg IV.

At 10:00 AM she was given Protonix 40 mg IV push and she signed consent for surgery. When she signed the consent for surgery, she had to write her understanding of the reason why she was having surgery. She wrote, "there is fluid on my heart, pressure on my ventricle".

Chapter 6

Courtney's Surgery

Courtney and I were very scared. I tried not to let my fear show in order to be strong for her. At 10:15 AM they took her to the operating room (OR), and she had a subxiphoid pericardial window to drain 150 mL's of clear yellow fluid in the pericardium of her heart and a 19 French Jackson-Pratt (JP) drain was placed. The cardiac surgeon had to put the drain in because she was not able to drain all the fluid off. She did not want to take more time in surgery than necessary because her blood pressure was so low.

According to medical records, they ran Lactated Ringers (LR) through her IV during surgery at 30 ml/hr. At 11:45 she was given Zofran 2 ml via IV. At 11:50 she was given neostigmine (neuromuscular blocking) 2 ml and glycopyrrolate (anticholinergic to reduce secretions in her airway) 2 ml via IV.

According to records, in the OR she was given lidocaine (anesthetic) 1 ml and versed (sedative) 2 ml's x3 separate doses. Courtney said the reason why it was three separate doses is because the anesthesiologist had a hard time getting her to go to sleep. She stated that he did his usual routine of preparing for

71

surgery. Then he gave her the first dose and continued his usual routine of preparing his equipment. He then asked her if she was sleepy and she said no. He gave her the second dose. After a while, he looked at the clock and asked, "Are you getting sleepy yet?" She said no. But then, after she thought about it, she said, "Well, maybe a little." After looking at the clock, he told her that they should be doing the surgery already and he admitted to her that according to her weight, he was not supposed to give her anymore. However, they could not operate until she was asleep. He gave her the third dose and she said that she still had to work on going to sleep. Before she fell asleep, he told her, "I'm pretty much just sitting here waiting for you to go to sleep." A short time after that, she had to close her eyes and help herself to relax in order to fall asleep.

We later learned the reason why it took a higher dose was because her brain was so poisoned. Vaccines are neurotoxins. More on the ingredients of vaccines later.

They also gave her dexamethasone (corticosteroid) 1 ml, rocuronium (muscle relaxer) 1 ml, etomidate (sedative) 7 ml, succinylcholine (muscle relaxer) 6 ml, Ancef (prophylactic antibiotic) 10 ml, and fentanyl (pain) (often given with anesthesia) 50 mcg/ml via IV.

At noon, her HR was recorded in the recovery room to be 90 with BP of 103/62, RR 23 and O2 sat 100% with a face shield and an oxygen flow rate of 15. At 12:05 it was charted that she was on a full-face mask at 15 L and her O2 sat was 100%. It was charted that she was anxious and restless, and her RR was 23. She was given 50 mcg/ml of fentanyl and versed 2mg/2ml.

At 12:10 PM they continued the LR and infused 400 ml's of it and changed it to sodium chloride 0.9% (NS) and infused 400 ml's of it. She was also given fentanyl 50 mcg/ml for a pain level of 10.

At 12:15 her MAP was 73, HR 78, RR 16 and she was wearing an oxygen mask with O2 sat of 100%. At 12:20 her MAP was 73, HR 68, RR 29 and O2 sat 100%. At 12:25 her MAP was 70, BP 102/58, HR 70, RR 33 and O2 sat 100%. It was charted that her eyes were closed, and she was resting quietly. However, it was also charted that she had a pain level of 8.

At 12:30 they called me and told me that she was in recovery and in satisfactory condition. Her HR was recorded in recovery at 94, BP 91/56, MAP 76, RR 33 and she was wearing an oxygen mask with an O2 sat of 100%. According to her medical records, they had to put her on a full-face mask at 5 L and her O2 sat was 100% but she was still having breathing difficulty. She was given fentanyl 50 mcg/ml for a pain level of 8.

At 12:40 she was given more fentanyl 50 mcg/ml for a pain level of 5 and her MAP was 69, BP 95/55, HR 84, RR 31 and O2 sat 100%. Courtney stated that her pain was in her upper abdomen. It was charted that her pain was aggravated with movement.

At 12:45 her MAP was 64, BP 89/50, HR 82, RR 37 and O2 sat 100%. At 12:50 her MAP was 66, BP 88/53, HR 78, RR 42 and O2 sat 100%. At 12:55 her MAP was 70, BP 94/56, HR 76, RR 42 and O2 sat 100%. At 12:57 her MAP was 68, BP 91/51, HR 76, RR 39 and O2 sat 100%.

Courtney does not remember wearing a full-face mask. She only remembers wearing a nasal cannula.

After surgery, she needed oxygen to maintain an oxygen saturation of greater than 90%. According to her medical records, while she was in recovery, they had a hard time getting her left ventricle to pick back up and her oxygen level started going down. They put her on oxygen and placed an arterial line to give her a Dopamine drip 400 mg [2mcg/kg/min] +premix D5W 250 ml.

At 1:00 PM they came to the surgery waiting room and informed me that they were going to have to transfer her to the intensive care unit (ICU) and they would show me to the waiting room. I was concerned because we expected her to go back to the room where she came from prior to surgery. I was getting nervous about what I was going to see after getting to her new room.

According to records, while still in recovery, the fentanyl had brought her pain level down to a 4 in her upper abdomen. Her MAP was 65, HR 90, RR 32 and O2 sat 100%. At 1:10 her MAP was 68, BP 91/55, HR 110, RR 31 and O2 sat 100%. At 1:15 her MAP was 75, HR 102, RR 31 and O2 sat 100%. At 1:20 her MAP was 72, BP 96/59, HR 100, RR 21 and O2 sat 100% via nasal cannula at 3 liters.

The doctor's orders were: "If temp is greater than 100.5 F, HR greater than 120 or less than 60, SBP greater than 180 or less than 90, RR greater than 26 or less than 12, or O2 sat less than 92 notify me. Titrate the drip to keep systolic bp equal or greater than 90 or mean equal or greater than 60."

Her arterial line read heart rate (HR) 103 and BP 91/58 and arterial BP 87/58.

At 1:45 they transferred her to the surgical intensive care unit (SICU). The JP drain had already drained out 20 mL's. During surgery, the cardiac surgeon sent off a fungus culture of the pericardial fluid which after five days was negative. Gram stain was also negative and anaerobic culture was negative after two days.

While reading medical records for this writing this book, the cytology pathology report read- "Final diagnosis: A) Pericardial fluid, cytology: Background of mixed inflammatory cells, predominantly lymphocytes, and occasional mesothelial cells. B) Pericardium, biopsy: Mesothelial lined fibromuscular tissue with minimal chronic inflammation."

What this means is there was chronic inflammation in the mesothelial lining of her pericardium, the sac around her heart. This chronic inflammation caused the pericardial effusion, which when left alone, prompted a pericardial window.

Chapter 7

Surgical Intensive Care Unit

When family and I walked into her critical care room, I was taken by surprise. Courtney was wearing oxygen via nasal cannula. She had a Dopamine drip and she seemed to be struggling to breath. The nurse informed me that her blood pressure and oxygen level started dropping while she was in surgery and again in recovery. While I was in the room with Courtney her breathing seemed to calm down.

At 2:00 PM the nurse charted "All nail beds are pale but warm extremities. Breath sounds in left lower, right middle and right lower lobes are diminished. She is wearing nasal cannula at 3L with O2 sat of 100%." She was given morphine 4 mg/ml for a pain level of 10. Her mean arterial pressure was 76, BP 98/59, HR 88 and RR 26.

At 2:10, she weighed 86.6 pounds! She had gained 4 ounces! Her total weight gain was 3.6 pounds! Her BMI was 14.87.

At 2:30 the Morphine was effective! At 3:00 the nurse charted "All nail beds are pale, but extremities are warm. Breath sounds in left lower, right middle and right lower lobes are diminished. She is wearing nasal cannula at 3L with O2 sat of 100%. Her PO intake less than

50% of normal in last 3 days." Her mean arterial pressure was 67, BP 98/58, HR 103 and RR 25. She rated her pain at a 10.

At 3:30 PM she felt like she needed to urinate. Her nurse placed her on a bedpan, but she was unable urinate. Her nurse inserted a urinary catheter and got out a bladder full!

At 4:20 she was given Zofran 4 mg/2 ml via IV for nausea.

At 4:45 her cardiologist came in and told me that she tested positive for tuberculosis (TB), but her chest x-ray was normal, indicating either acute or latent infection and an infectious disease doctor had been assigned to her case. The JP drain had drained out 20 mL's.

At 4:50 the Zofran was effective! At 5:00 she was given Morphine 4 mg/ml for a pain level of 10.

At 5:15 the nurse was notified by the cardiologist that the TB test was positive, and an infectious disease doctor was notified. The cardiologist explained that the infectious disease doctor stated that it was not necessary to place her on contact precautions.

At 6:05 her Lactated Ringers (LR) bag was changed, and she was given Morphine 4mg/ml for a pain level of 10. At 6:45 the morphine was effective! At 7 her nurse charted all nail beds were pale, but extremities were warm. Breath sounds in left lower, right middle and right lower lobes were diminished. She was wearing nasal cannula at 3L with an O2 sat of 99%. She was experiencing nausea.

Her infectious disease doctor charted one of her problems was abnormal loss of weight. He initiated a care plan of positive QuantiFERON-TB gold test.

At 7:15 PM she was given Tramadol 50 mg tab for a pain level of 10. At 7:50 she was given sucralfate 10 ml. Her mean arterial pressure was 60, BP 88/52, HR 91, RR 45 and O2 sat 99% via nasal cannula at 3 liters.

At 8:15 the Tramadol had lowered her pain level to a 4. At 9:00 her mean arterial pressure was 67, BP 88/52, HR 100, RR 32 and O2 sat 99% via NC at 3 liters. At 9:23 she was given Tylenol 650 mg tabs, sodium chloride nasal spray and Zofran 4mg/2 ml. At 9:53 the Zofran was effective!

At 10:05 she was given Morphine for a pain level of 7. Her mean arterial pressure was 64, BP 82/54, HR 98, RR 28 and O2 sat 99%. At 10:23 the Tylenol was not effective. She still had a pain level of 5. At 10:35 the Morphine had lowered her pain to a 1.

At 11:00 her infectious disease doctor came and did a consult. I informed him that she had no documented exposure to TB. She had worked in daycare and retail. She had been unemployed for the last 4 or 5 months. She had been experiencing shortness of breath, palpitations, and some difficulty swallowing solids and liquids. He treated her as latent TB and gave her Isoniazid prophylactically. He added to her lab order an acid-fast bacillus stain and culture on the pathology that was already sent to the lab. He said there was no need for isolation because her chest x-ray showed no consolidation.

The nurse charted all nail beds were pale, but extremities were warm. Breath sounds in left lower lobe and right middle and lower lobes were diminished using nasal cannula at 3L with 99% saturation. She was experiencing nausea. Her mean arterial pressure was 61, BP 80/52, HR 97 and RR 24. Her input was recorded as 4,163.54 ml's and output 3,105 ml's.

April 9, at midnight her mean arterial pressure was 51, BP 76/44, HR 89, RR 47 and O2 sat 99% via NC at 3L. At 12:45 AM the doctor ordered an NS bolus. At 2:30 her mean arterial pressure was 51, BP 72/44, HR 91, RR 34 and O2 sat 100%. At 2:45 her mean arterial pressure was 51, BP 77/45, HR 88, RR 45 and O2 sat 100%.

At 3:00 AM the nurse charted all nail beds were pale, but extremities were warm. Left lower lobe and right middle and lower lobes were diminished. She notified the doctor that her blood pressure was trending down. She was also experiencing nausea. I was becoming concerned again and getting scared.

The doctor ordered another 500 ml stat NS bolus to get her BP up. Her mean arterial pressure was 56, BP 84/48, HR 82 and RR 48.

Her MPV was low at 7.0 and chloride was high but better at 112.

A low MPV count does increase the risk for serious blood loss if you are injured. It is often due to inflammatory conditions in the body and can cause anemia. Therefore, Courtney's heart was inflamed, and she was probably anemic (low iron).

At 3:10 it was charted that her blood pressure was trending down. Her physician was notified, and orders received. At 3:15 she was given Tramadol 50 mg tab for a pain level of 8 and her mean arterial pressure was 56, BP 79/50, HR 87, RR 20 and O2 sat 100%.

At 3:30 her MAP was 59, BP 78/47, HR 87, RR 31 and O2 sat 99%. At 3:45 her mean arterial pressure was 59, BP 82/48, HR 87, RR 31 and O2 sat 99%. At 4:00 her mean arterial pressure was 58, BP 83/47, HR 89, RR 49 and O2 sat 99% via NC at 3L. At 4:15 the Tramadol had brought her pain level down to a 2 and her mean arterial pressure was 53, BP 75/43, HR 89, RR 19 and O2 sat 99%.

At 4:30 AM her mean arterial pressure was 54, BP 77/44, HR 89, RR 19 and O2 sat 99%. At 4:45 her mean arterial pressure was 57, BP 81/46, HR 84, RR 46 and O2 sat 99% via 3L NC. At 5:00 the JP drain put out 10 mL's and her mean arterial pressure was 54, BP 77/45, HR 88, RR 29 and O2 sat 99%.

At 7:00 the nurse charted that all nail beds were pale, and breath sounds in left lower lobe, and right middle and lower lobe were diminished. She was on nasal cannula with 100% saturation and extremities were pale and warm and her skin was pale. Her mean arterial pressure was 56, BP 87/48, HR 89 and RR 17. Courtney rated her pain at an 8.

At 7:30 her doctor came in and ordered an auto differential and CBC with differential. She was given a 500 ml NS bolus. At 8:15 she was given Tramadol 50 mg tab for a pain level of 10 and Zofran 4 mg/2 ml for nausea. At 8:44 the Zofran was effective!

At 9:00, her cardiologist reported the rub had resolved! In other words, while listening to her heart with his stethoscope, he no longer heard the pericardial effusion. Taking the fluid off her heart was successful! And, another 50 mL's of fluid had drained off her heart and had been sent to the lab. However, she was still experiencing hypotension (low blood pressure) while on a Dopamine drip (Dopamine/D5W 400 mg [2 mcg/kg/min] +premix D5W 250 ml @ 2.95 mL/hr. Her doctor thought her blood pressure was low because of pain meds. His target was a systolic blood pressure of 95. He ordered an NS bolus to help get her BP up and magnesium sulfate 8 ml with 50 ml NS IV. He wrote for more labs such as a BMP (basic metabolic profile) and CBC (complete blood count).

She was given Zoloft 25 mg tab, Protonix 40 mg tab, multivitamin 1 tab, Indocin 50 mg/2 caps, Colchicine 0.6 mg tab, sodium chloride nasal spray, and Carafate 10 ml. I did not realize after the surgery that he still had her on Colchicine. If I had known, I would have requested that it be stopped.

At 9:27 AM the Tramadol had brought her pain level down to a 3. At 9:45 AM the magnesium sulfate was started. At 10:00 her mean arterial pressure was 56, HR 85, BP 98/52, RR 44 and O2 sat 99%.

At 10:41 she was given Phenergan 25 mg tab. The nurse charted at 11:00 that all nail beds were pale, but extremities were warm, and her skin was pale. She was drowsy and weak. She had a pain level of 8.

At 11:15 she was given Morphine 4 mg/ml for a pain level of 10. Her RR were 18. At 11:45 the Morphine and Phenergan were effective!

At noon, the cardiac surgeon came in and she was mad because Courtney was so "sedated" that she was unable to accurately assess her.

First, it took an increased amount of anesthesia to put her to sleep for surgery. Second, her nurse was giving her Morphine (pain) and Phenergan (nausea). The cardiac surgeon complained that the meds were making her unstable because she was too sedated. She discontinued both!

I was so mad because Courtney was finally getting some much-needed rest! Courtney's nurse told me that was the way she was! They said she was a great surgeon but had a short temper. She ordered Reglan (nausea) but nothing for pain!

Her mean arterial pressure was 48, BP 95/46, HR 75, RR 27 and O2 sat 99%. At 12:15 PM she was given Zofran 2 ml via IV for nausea. At 12:45 the Zofran was effective!

At 1:30 PM her cardiac surgeon came back and discontinued the bladder foley and wrote for Courtney's magnesium level to be checked and ordered Toradol (pain).

At 1:53 she was given Indocin 50 mg/2 caps, Carafate 10 ml and Tramadol 50 mg tab for a pain level of 5. At 2:00 her RR was 29, BP 110/59 and O2 sat 100%.

The nurse charted at 3:00 that Courtney was pale, her sensory perception was slightly limited, her mobility was slightly limited, and she was weak. She was given Reglan 2 ml for nausea and Toradol for a pain level of 10.

At 3:15 her doctor came in and Courtney denied shortness of breath! Praise God!

Her nurse charted that she was a nutrition risk due to decreased intake because of nausea and vomiting from severe GERD. She was placed on a 1409-1537 kcal/d diet. Her nail bed color on her hands and feet were pale. The nurse charted that her left lower, right middle and right lower lobes were diminished. She was receiving oxygen via nasal cannula at 100%. Her extremities were pale but warm. At 3:30 the Reglan was effective!

At 3:34 PM her nurse charted, "Per mother, pt. usually weighs about 110 pounds. Pt going through divorce currently and husband was buying video games, so there was no money for food, which is part of the reason pt. was losing weight. The second reason for the weight loss was d/t severe GERD. Pt would get nauseated with eating. Pt currently lives with mom. Mom reports setting up with the Wyatt clinic and getting food stamps. Mom states pt. having a dietician consult at the end of this month at the Wyatt clinic. Will try full liquids for dinner and advance as tolerated to a regular diet, per mom. Eats mostly bland foods d/t GERD. Does not eat spicy foods or carbonated beverages. Did not tolerate breakfast this morning. Ate lunch and was tolerated. Appetite poor, N/V."

At 3:52 PM her nurse charted her plan of care as nutrition deficit. She was consuming a clear liquid diet and meeting 50% of her estimated needs.

At 4:00 her mean arterial pressure was 69, BP 97/56, HR 113, RR 18 and O2 sat 100%. At

4:30 the Toradol was effective! At 5:00 the JP drained 40 ml's and her mean arterial pressure was 68, BP 100/51, HR 71, RR 45 and O2 sat 99%.

At 5:45 she was given Zofran 4 mg/2 ml, Carafate 10 ml, and Indocin 50 mg/2 caps. At 6:00 her mean arterial pressure was 69, BP 98/55, HR 94, RR 34 and O2 sat 99%. At 6:30 she was given Tramadol 50 mg tab for a pain level of 10 and the Zofran was effective. At 7:00 she was on a clear liquid diet and her mean arterial pressure was 67, BP 94/52, HR 74, RR 50 and O2 sat 100% via NC at 2 L. At 7:30 the Tramadol was effective! At 8:00 her mean arterial pressure was 78, HR 79, RR 48 and O2 sat 99%. At 8:15 she was given Carafate 10 ml and sodium chloride nasal spray.

At 8:30 PM the arterial line read HR 82, ABP 108/64. A nursing plan of care of ineffective airway clearance and total self-care deficit was initiated.

At 9:00 her mean arterial pressure was 72, HR 71, BP 99/57, RR 37 and O2 sat 100%. At 9:50 she was given Toradol 1 ml for a pain level of 8. Her mean arterial pressure was 66, BP 92/53, HR 73, RR 46 and O2 sat 95%. At 11:00 she was given Zofran 4 mg/2 ml and it was charted that her nail bed color was pale. Her mean arterial pressure was 66, BP 93/54, HR100, RR 22 and O2 sat 95% on RA. Her intake was recorded as 4,064 ml's and output 4,930 ml's.

April 10 at midnight her mean arterial pressure was 70, BP 101/55, HR 72, RR 42 and O2 sat 95%. Her monocytes were low at 0.12. Monocytes are a white blood cell that help the body to fight off infections. A low number of monocytes, called monocytopenia, is the result of a decrease in the overall level of white blood cells.

At 1:00 AM her mean arterial pressure was 71, BP 104/56, HR 86, RR 22 and O2 sat 96%. At 2:00 her mean arterial pressure was 65, BP 90/52, HR 77, RR 32 and O2 sat 95%. At 2:30 the Toradol and Zofran were effective! The Toradol brought her pain level down to a 3. At 3:00 her mean arterial pressure was 63, BP 90/49, HR 77, RR 46 and O2 sat 96% on RA. At 4:00 her mean arterial pressure was 63, BP 90/50, HR 88, RR 16 and O2 sat 96%. At 4:30 her arterial line read HR 90 and ABP 100/54. At 5:00 AM the JP drained out 40 ml's.

Her infectious disease doctor ordered a chest x-ray to check for congestion. She was given Zofran 2 ml and Toradol 1 ml for a pain level of 7. Her mean arterial pressure was 70,

BP 97/55, HR 84, RR 35 and O2 sat 97%. At
5:40 AM the Zofran was effective and the
Toradol had brought her pain level down to a 2.
At 6:00 her mean arterial pressure was 64, BP
91/50, HR 83, RR 18 and O2 sat 96%.

At 6:50 the arterial line read HR 91 and ABP
87/48. She was drowsy and her speech was
slowed but clear and another chest x-ray was
done.

At 7:50 her doctor ordered Ensure with
breakfast, lunch and dinner. Her mean arterial
pressure was 68, BP 90/57, HR 107, RR 35 and
O2 sat 97%. Her nurse charted that her arterial
line was in her left radial. Courtney was pale.
She had a JP drain in her left chest that was
draining via suction.

At 8:15 AM her mean arterial pressure was
75, HR 139, RR 21 and O2 sat 99%. At 8:30
her mean arterial pressure was 72, HR 115, RR
16 and O2 sat 97%.

At 8:42 she was given Colchicine 0.6 mg
tab, sodium chloride nasal spray, Zoloft 25 mg
tab, MiraLAX 17 gm, Protonix 40 mg tab,
multivitamin 1 tab, Indocin 50 mg/2 caps,
Tramadol 50 mg tab for a pain level of 8, Zofran
2 ml and Carafate 10 ml. Her mean arterial
pressure was 84, HR 138, RR 20 and O2 sat

98%. At 9:00 her mean arterial pressure was 65, BP 84/54, HR 108, RR 25 and O2 sat 96%.

At 9:15, her nurse charted Zofran was effective, but it was not because when her NP came in Courtney was experiencing an episode of GERD that included dry heaves. Thankfully, she denied chest pain.

The JP drain put out 80 mL's in the last 24 hours. She was still on the Dopamine drip and they increased the dose to 15 mcg. I was getting concerned that her right ventricle was not going to pick up. I stood at the foot of her bed and I prayed over her "Lord, please save my daughter."

The NP decided to order a cortisol level. The order read "please call if cortisol level abnormal, wean drip for SBP => 90." Her mean arterial pressure was 72, BP 100/59, HR 96, RR 37 and O2 sat 97%.

At 9:50 the Tramadol had brought her pain level down to a 1. Her mean arterial pressure was 69, BP 94/58, HR 118, RR 28 and O2 sat 97%. At 10:45 she was started on sodium chloride 0.9% (NS) via IV and her mean arterial pressure was 68, BP 93/55, HR 89, RR 29 and O2 sat 97%. At 11:00 she was drowsy, and her mean arterial pressure was 69, BP 93/57, HR 102, RR 19 and O2 sat 97%. At 11:30 her mean arterial pressure was 71, BP 96/58, HR 91, RR 32 and O2 sat 97%.

At 12:45 PM her mean arterial pressure was 55, BP 72/46, HR 128, RR 23 and O2 sat 97%. At 1:00 she was given magnesium oxide 400 mg tab, Mylanta 30 ml, Carafate 10 ml, and Indocin 50 mg/2 caps. Her mean arterial pressure was 67, BP 87/56, HR 115, RR 20 and O2 sat 98%. At 1:15 she was given Zofran 2 ml and her mean arterial pressure was 74, HR 122, RR 32 and O2 sat 98%.

At 1:30 her cardiac surgeon ordered to discontinue the urinary foley and decrease IV to 50 cc/hr. At 1:50 the Zofran was effective, and her mean arterial pressure was 78, HR 101, RR 15 and O2 sat 97%.

At 2:35 her doctor came in and her nurse reported to him that Courtney had another GERD episode after lunch. Praise God, she denied shortness of breath! He wrote an order for Phenergan and magnesium oxide.

Do you remember her cardiac surgeon discontinuing the Phenergan?

At 2:45 PM the arterial line read HR 134, ABP 141/85, mean arterial pressure was 86, RR 23, O2 sat 100% and she was given Toradol 1 ml for a pain level of 9. At 3:00 her mean arterial pressure was 68, BP 91/56, HR 104, RR 14 and O2 sat 100%. At 3:15 the Toradol had brought her pain level down to a 2 and her mean arterial pressure was 66, BP 94/53, HR 95, RR 15 and O2 sat 98%.

At 3:16 Courtney had an EKG change called ventricular bigeminy.

Ventricular bigeminy is an abnormal heart rhythm. Ventricular bigeminy might be a sign that the heart is in distress. It is a sign that some abnormal process is occurring in the body and causing harm. Her cardiologist was notified but no new orders were received. I was so thankful that what her heart had been doing at home was finally being recorded.

At 4:00 it was charted that her breath sounds were diminished, and she was drowsy. While writing this book, Courtney's medical records showed that she had a urinary catheter. However, her cardiac surgeon ordered it to be removed and it was removed. In other words, at this point, Courtney did not have a urinary catheter.

At 4:30 PM her mean arterial pressure was 62, BP 86/49, HR 85, RR 17 and O2 sat 96%. At 5:00 the JP drain put out 50 ml's. At 5:15 her mean arterial pressure was 71, BP 96/59, HR 90, RR 27 and O2 sat 98%. At 5:30 she was given Zofran 2 ml and Carafate 10 ml. At 5:45 her mean arterial pressure was 70, BP 94/57, HR 87, RR 29 and O2 sat 97%.

At 6:00 the Zofran was not effective. She had two IV's, one was NS, and the other was a Dopamine drip.

At 6:45 PM her mean arterial pressure was 70, BP 94/58, HR 85, RR 26 and O2 sat 97%. At 7:00 her mean arterial pressure was 69, BP 93/56, HR 84, RR 39 and O2 sat 97% on RA.

It was charted that she was bedfast, and her mobility was slightly limited. Her nutrition was probably inadequate, she was drowsy, and she had a weak gait. While writing this book, I also noticed her nurse charted PO (by mouth) intake less than 50% of normal in last three days.

At 7:15 she was given Phenergan 1 ml and her mean arterial pressure was 71, BP 93/59, HR 93, RR 15 and O2 sat 96%. At 7:30 her mean arterial pressure was 80, HR 102, RR 29 and O2 sat 97%. At 8:00 her mean arterial pressure was 73, HR 87, RR 13 and O2 sat 96%. At 9:15 PM her mean arterial pressure was 67, BP 88/56, HR 88, RR 26 and O2 sat 97%. At 10:00 her mean arterial pressure was 66, BP 84/56, HR 122, RR 19 and O2 sat 98%. At 10:15 her mean arterial pressure was 64, BP 86/52, HR 80, RR 14 and O2 sat 96%. At 11:30

her mean arterial pressure was 67, BP 94/52, HR 77, RR 32 and O2 sat 97%. At 11:45 her mean arterial pressure was 65, BP 92/50, HR 74, RR 16 and O2 sat 97%.

Her intake was recorded as 2,519 ml's and output 2,780 ml's.

April 11 at midnight her mean arterial pressure was 66, BP 94/51, HR 73, RR 32 and O2 sat 97%. At 1:00 AM the arterial line read HR 77, ABP 85/47, mean arterial pressure 63, RR 21 and O2 sat 96%.

At 2:15 she was given Phenergan 1 ml and Toradol 1 ml for a pain level of 5. Her mean arterial pressure was 71, BP 99/57, HR 83, RR 17 and O2 sat 97%.

At 2:45 the Toradol had brought her pain level down to a 3. At 4:30 her mean arterial pressure was 64, BP 93/49, HR 82, RR 28 and O2 sat 97%. At 4:45 her arterial pressure was 69, BP 95/54, HR 76, RR 21 and O2 sat 98%.

At 5:00 the JP drained out 30 ml's. At 5:15 her mean arterial pressure was 54, BP 80/40, HR 72, RR 12 and O2 sat 96%. At 5:45 her mean arterial pressure was 57, BP 85/43, HR 76, RR 20 and O2 sat 96%.

At 7:00 her nurse charted that Courtney had been threatened or physically hurt in the past

12 months and that there was evidence of abuse or neglect. It was charted that Courtney was weak in all extremities. She had two twenty-gauge IV's, one in her left forearm and the other in her right forearm.

At 9:00 she was given MiraLAX 17 gm, Protonix 40 mg tab, multivitamin 1 tab, magnesium oxide 400 mg tab, Indocin 50 mg/2 tabs, Colchicine 0.6 mg tab, Phenergan 1 ml, Carafate 10 ml, sodium chloride nasal spray, Zoloft 25 mg tab and Toradol 1 ml for a pain level of 5. Her BP was 94/57, HR 73, RR 25 and O2 sat 99%.

At 9:30 the Toradol was effective! At 10:00 her BP was 83/47, HR 59, RR 24 and O2 sat 100%. At 10:30 she was given Buspar (anti-anxiety) 5 mg tab. At 11:00 her BP was 80/52, HR 61, RR 23 and O2 sat 98%.

At noon, her BP was 92/50, HR 63, RR 29 and O2 sat 97%.

At 12:40 her cardiologist came in and Courtney stated that she does not feel good, however she was not having much pain. Her hypotension had not changed. He thought the reason for her hypotension was the Dopamine drip.

Does this make any sense? The Dopamine drip was supposed to help increase her blood pressure, not decrease it!

He stated that Courtney's cortisol level was "within normal range". He was going to order physical therapy/occupational therapy evaluation for generalized strengthening and progressive ambulation (walking). He wanted to wean the Dopamine for systolic blood pressure of greater than 90.

At 1:00 PM she was given Tramadol 50 mg tab for a pain level of 4, Zofran 2 ml, Carafate 10 ml, and Indocin 50 mg/2 caps. Her RR was 26, BP 97/58, HR 71 and O2 sat 98%.

At 2:30 her doctor came in and Courtney was complaining that she was not feeling good and she was experiencing nausea. Yet, her nurse charted that the Zofran was effective. Huh? Her nurse also charted barriers to learning due to acuity of illness.

At 3:00 Courtney was drowsy. At 5:14 she was given Carafate 10 ml and Indocin 50 mg/2 caps. At 6:00 the JP drained out 30 ml's and she was given Phenergan 1 ml and Toradol 1ml for a pain level of 4. At 7:00 she was experiencing nausea and the Toradol was effective.

At 8:15 her mean arterial pressure was 59, BP 84/46, HR 76, RR 14 and O2 sat 96%. At 8:30 her mean arterial pressure was 67, BP 91/54, HR 91, RR 16 and O2 sat 96%.

At 8:45 she was given Tums 500 mg tab, Carafate 10 ml, and Zofran 2 ml's. At 9:00 she was given magnesium oxide 400 mg tab, and Tramadol 50 mg tab for a pain level of 7. The Zofran was charted as effective and her mean arterial pressure was 60, BP 84/46, HR 75, RR 24 and O2 sat 96%.

At 9:15 her mean arterial pressure was 71, HR 106, RR 28 and O2 sat 97%. At 9:45 her mean arterial pressure was 69, BP 93/57, HR 74, RR 16 and O2 sat 96%.

At 10:00 the Tramadol was effective. At 11:00 she was experiencing nausea and drowsiness and her mean arterial pressure was 64, BP 88/51, HR 74, RR 13 and O2 sat 96%. At 11:30 her mean arterial pressure was 70, BP 93/57, HR 86, RR 22 and O2 sat 97%.

Her intake was recorded as 1,837 ml's and output 940 ml's.

April 12 at midnight her mean arterial pressure was 63, BP 87/51, HR 78, RR 13 and O2 sat 97%. At 1:00 AM the arterial line read HR 72, ABP 85/47, mean arterial pressure was

64, RR 16 and O2 sat 97%. At 1:30 her mean arterial pressure was 64, BP 90/51, HR 69, RR 11 and O2 sat 97%.

At 2:30 she was given Phenergan 1 ml and Toradol 1 ml for a pain level of 5. At 3:00 the Toradol had brought her pain level down to a 2 and she was complaining of nausea.

At 3:30 her mean arterial pressure was 64, BP 86/53, HR 84, RR 11 and O2 sat 96%. At 4:15 her mean arterial pressure was 59, BP 81/48, HR 78, RR 11 and O2 sat 96%. At 4:45 her mean arterial pressure was 63, BP 90/50, HR 86, RR 19 and O2 sat 97%. At 5:45 her mean arterial pressure was 58, BP 81/46, HR 84, RR 39 and O2 sat 96%.

At 6:00 AM the JP drained out 10 ml's and her mean arterial pressure was 53, BP 77/42, HR 78, RR 15 and O2 sat 96%. I was getting scared again. I stood at the foot of her bed and prayed, "Lord, please save my daughter."

At 6:15 her mean arterial pressure was 56, BP 81/44, HR 76, RR 21 and O2 sat 96%.

She weighed 86.4 pounds. She had lost two ounces.

At 7:00 she was experiencing tachycardia of 110, complaining of fatigue and experiencing shortness of breath with an O2 sat of 98% on room air. Her mean arterial pressure was 59, BP 85/46 and RR 19.

At 7:15 AM her mean arterial pressure was 61, BP 88/47, HR 79, RR 18 and O2 sat 97%. At 7:30 her mean arterial pressure was 64, BP 90/50, HR 83, RR 15 and O2 sat 97%. At 8:00 her mean arterial pressure was 53, BP 76/41, HR 93, RR 21 and O2 sat 100%.

At 8:15 she was given Phenergan 0.5 ml and Toradol 1 ml for a pain level of 8. Her mean arterial pressure was 75, BP 109/57, HR 80, RR 29 and O2 sat 100%. At 8:30 the Toradol had lowered her pain level down to a 3. Since she was still having pain, she was given Carafate 10 ml and Protonix 40 mg tab. Her mean arterial pressure was 65, BP 96/51, HR 98, RR 36 and O2 sat 100%. At 8:45 her mean arterial pressure was 67, BP 96/53, HR 99, RR 21, O2 sat 100% and her pain level was a 3.

An on-call doctor came in Courtney's room while she was asleep, and he had a shocked look on his face. He admitted to me that he expected to see an elderly person lying in the bed, not a young person. He said, "I want to let you know that I have spent the past hour looking through her chart, I hope you don't mind. I think it is safe for me to admit that we have no idea what we are doing with her. Her condition has me puzzled. I am going to pray for her." He asked me if I was keeping a journal of what was going on with her. I said, "No. I just want my daughter well again." He said, "You might want to consider writing a book in the future. I will be interested to know how this turns out." He wished me the best and left her room. I never saw him again. I do hope he reads this book.

At 9:00 AM she was given Zoloft 25 mg tab, multivitamin 1 tab, magnesium oxide 400 mg tab, Indocin 50 mg/2 caps, and Colchicine 0.6 mg tab. Her mean arterial pressure was 46, BP 70/36, HR 106, RR 23 and O2 sat 100%. I was getting concerned again.

At 9:15 her MAP was 66, BP 92/58, HR 99, RR 20 and O2 sat 100%. At 9:30 her MAP was 66, BP 92/58, HR 109, RR 36 and O2 sat 100%. At 9:45 her MAP was 72, HR 113, RR 23 and O2 sat 100%.

At 10:00 her cardiologist came in and Courtney said she was feeling ok, but she had a rough night. The Dopamine drip had to be increased to 18 mcg/kg/min. He decided to taper the Indocin. He was thinking about trying Fluorinef.

Fluorinef is a man-made (synthetic) form of a glucocorticoid that is made by the body.

Glucocorticoid is a hormone. It is used to treat low glucocorticoid levels caused by disease of the adrenal gland. Glucocorticoids are needed in many ways for the body to function well. They are important for salt and water balance and keeping blood pressure normal.

A nursing care plan of ineffective airway clearance was initiated. At 10:20 her nurse charted barriers to learning due to acuity of illness. At 10:30 she was given Zofran 2 ml and Tramadol 50 mg tab for a pain level of 7. Her MAP was 64, BP 97/54, HR 90, RR 18 and O2 sat 96%.

At 11:00 AM she was experiencing shortness of breath with an O2 sat of 98% on room air. It was charted that the Zofran was effective! At 11:30 the Tramadol had lowered her pain level down to a 2 and her MAP was 77, HR 88, RR 29 and O2 sat 96%. At 11:45 her MAP was 70, HR 97, RR 23 and O2 sat 96%.

At noon, her MAP was 59, BP 79/52, HR 102, RR 28 and O2 sat 97%. At 12:30 she was given Carafate 10 ml. At 12:45 her MAP was 71, HR 77, RR 20 and O2 sat 98%. At 1:15 her MAP was 57, BP 89/49, HR 103, RR 20 and O2 sat 99%.

At 1:30 PM her doctor came in and Courtney was experiencing nausea. Her potassium level had gone down again to 3.3. Her nurse was replacing it per protocol. Her doctor mentioned again to try Fluorinef and said we may need to do another echo. He wrote an order for Morphine to control her pain and for lab to check her magnesium level.

Do you remember that her cardiac surgeon took her off the Morphine?

Courtney's magnesium was low, so it was replaced per protocol. She was also having some nasal congestion, so he ordered some saline nasal spray. He also ordered a Basic Metabolic Panel (BMP) and a CBC.

At 1:45 PM she was given Mylanta 30 ml and her MAP was 70, HR 80, RR 24 and O2 sat 98%.

While writing this book and reviewing Courtney's medical records, I noticed that at 3:00 she was placed on "Notify Provider of SEVERE Sepsis Risk". If I would have known this while she was in the hospital, I would have insisted on more action being taken! It stated, "SIRS Criteria: HR (101 bpm), RR (30 br/min) Organ Dysfunction: (64 mmHg) Systolic BP (87 mmHg) Sepsis Alert: The following information suggests that this patient may have sepsis. Please ensure the patient is on the appropriate medication therapy. Early goal directed therapy is essential for the treatment of sepsis. Time dependent intervention may impact patient outcome."

Courtney was complaining of fatigue, shortness of breath with an O2 sat of 95% on room air and experiencing sinus tachycardia at 104. She was given Phenergan 0.5 ml and Tramadol 50 mg for a pain level of 8.

At 2:00 her MAP was 69, BP 110/58, HR 106 and O2 sat 97%. At 3:00 her MAP was 64, BP 87/57, HR 101, RR 30, O2 sat 95% on RA and her pain level was an 8. At 3:45 her MAP was 63, BP 86/57, HR 104, RR 21 and O2 sat 96%. At 4:00 the Tramadol had brought her pain level down to a 3. At 4:45 her MAP was 60, BP 93/51, HR 79, RR 34 and O2 sat 97%. At 5:00 her MAP was 66, BP 97/57, HR 79, RR 19 and O2 sat 96% on RA.

At 6:00 the JP drained 30 ml's and she was given MiraLAX 17 gm, Zofran 2 ml, Toradol 1 ml for a pain level of 8, and Carafate 10 ml. Her MAP was 100, BP 120/93, HR 72, RR 45 and O2 sat 99%. At 6:50 the arterial line HR 84 and NBP was 110/72. At 7:20 she was given Mylanta 30 ml and her MAP was 78, HR 124 and O2 sat 96%. At 7:30 her MAP was 84, HR 73 and O2 sat 99%.

At 8:20 PM she was experiencing shortness of breath with an O2 sat of 100% on room air. At 8:30 she was given Mylicon 80 mg tab and Phenergan 0.5 ml. At 9:00 her MAP was 54, BP 72/48, HR 109 and O2 sat 94%. At 10:15 her MAP was 64, BP 89/58, HR 81 and O2 sat 96%.

Her intake was recorded as 3,191.5 ml's and output 4,000 ml's.

April 13, her WBCs were low but better at 3.7. At 12:15 AM she was experiencing shortness of breath with an O2 sat of 96%. Her MAP was 67, BP 97/57, and HR 81.

At 2:00 she was given Phenergan 0.5 ml and Toradol 1 ml for a pain level of 6 and her MAP was 67, BP 94/58, HR 68 and O2 sat 96%. At 2:30 the Toradol had brought her pain level down to a 2. At 3:15 her MAP was 56, BP 83/49, HR 76 and O2 sat 97%. At 3:30 her MAP was 67, BP 101/57, HR 79 and O2 sat 97%.

At 4:00 AM she was experiencing shortness of breath with an O2 sat of 96%, MAP was 68 and HR 75. At 4:30 her MAP was 54, BP 76/48, HR 86 and O2 sat 97%. At 4:45 her MAP was 65, BP 100/54, HR 75 and O2 sat 97%. At 5:00 the JP drained 20 ml's.

She weighed 90.6 pounds! She gained 4.2 pounds! Her total weight gain was 7.6 pounds!

At 7:00 her cardiologist came in and said Courtney no longer had right ventricle gallop or rub! However, her low blood pressure was persisting. He ordered another echo. He informed us he was considering a right heart cath if any echo abnormalities.

At 7:15 her MAP was 63, BP 88/55, HR 83 and O2 sat 97%. At 7:30 her arterial line HR was 98, NBP 101/67, MAP was 75, RR 24 and she was experiencing shortness of breath with an O2 sat of 96%. She was given Tramadol 50 mg tab for a pain level of 4 and Zofran 2 ml.

At 7:45 her MAP was 60, BP 85/54, HR 94 and O2 sat 98%.

At 8:00 AM her cardiac surgeon came in and ordered a Free T4 and Free T3. The Zofran was effective, and her MAP was 65, BP 98/55, HR 95 and O2 sat 99%. At 8:45 the Tramadol was effective, and she was given Colchicine 0.6 mg tab. At 8:45 she was given Zoloft 25 mg tab, MiraLAX 17 gm, multivitamin 1 tab, Protonix 40 mg tab, magnesium oxide 400 mg tab, Indocin 50 mg/2 caps, and Carafate 10 ml.

At 9:52 occupational therapy (OT) charted a "problem list" which included: abnormal loss of weight, acute pain, at risk for falls, at risk of pressure sore, bowel dysfunction, GERD, ineffective airway clearance, positive TB test, total self-care deficit, acute pericardial effusion, chest pain, cardiovascular and respiratory. OT charted "Pt with complicated cardiac history. Her HR went up to 130 with ambulation in hallway."

Courtney does NOT have a cardiac history! She did, however, have a complicated cardiac diagnosis.

At 10:02 AM physical therapy (PT) charted, "Pt is pleasant young female very motivated for therapy. Pt doing very well and may not require much therapy but due to medical complications, pt. requiring close monitoring of vital signs during ambulation at this time. Pt ambulating with quick, steady gait but require the assistance of either IV pole or HHA at this time. Pt denied pain or SOB; pt. just reported some nausea at the end of ambulation. Pt wanting to ambulate as much as possible. PT will continue to ambulate with pt. until pt. feels confident to ambulate on her own or with family especially while in ICU while pt. still requires monitoring. Pt has had low BP and has been unable to get off BP drip due to BP "bottoming out"."

At 10:00 her MAP was 65, BP 94/56, HR 89 and O2 sat 99%. Her nurse charted barriers to learning due to acuity of illness.

At 11:15 she was experiencing shortness of breath with an O2 sat of 98% on room air. She was given Phenergan 0.5 ml and Toradol 1 ml for a pain level of 8. At 11:30 her MAP was 62, BP 83/56, HR 93 and O2 sat 97%. At 11:45 she rated her pain at a 2.

At 11:50 her NP came in and Courtney was having chest pain, same as on admission but not as bad. She was still on 15 mcg of Dopamine. When the Dopamine was titrated down her systolic blood pressure dropped into the 70's. The arterial line HR 84 and NBP 103/66.

At noon, the echo was ordered due to persistent hypotension and unspecified tachycardia following pericardial window.

At 12:45 her MAP was 70, BP 101/59, HR 74 and O2 sat 97%. At 12:50 she was given Tramadol 50 mg tab for a pain level of 7, Zofran 2 ml, and Carafate 10 ml. Her RR was 22.

At 1:21 the Zofran was effective!

At 1:45 PM she had another echo done. At 2:45 she was experiencing severe GERD.

While writing this book I noticed her nurse charted "increased nutrient need, increased demand for nutrients. Recent weight loss of 10 pounds. Need for weight gain and recovery from surgery. Estimated energy needs, 1409-1537 kcal/d. Ensure chocolate with meals. Continue Ensure chocolate with meals to increase calorie and protein intake and elicit consistent weight gain. Next meal, diet type GI soft. Pt has gained weight since 4/9, approximately 4 pounds, could be partially fluid weight although pt. eating well now."

It was charted that her nutrition deficit nursing plan of care had been met because she was tolerating a soft diet and drinking Ensure with meals.

At 3:30 PM she was experiencing shortness of breath with an O2 sat of 97%, MAP 70, HR 100 and weakness. At 3:48 she was given Zofran 2 ml and Toradol 1 ml for a pain level of 4. At 4:00 her MAP was 66, BP 87/60, HR 90 and O2 sat 97%. At 4:15 her MAP was 68, BP 96/59, HR 83 and O2 sat 96%.

At 5:11 she was given Carafate 10 ml and her MAP was 61, BP 87/53, HR 81 and O2 sat 96%.

At 6:00 her doctor came in and we reported to him that Courtney had chest pain and her

MAP was 66, BP 94/59, HR 88 and O2 sat 98%. The JP drain put out 30 ml's. The echo resulted showing left ventricular ejection fraction of 55% to 60%. No clinically significant pericardial effusion. While writing this book, I noticed in her medical records that this echo also indicated possible left sided pleural effusion. I was never told about this.

At 6:15 PM she was given Mylanta 30 ml and Phenergan 0.5 ml. At 6:30 her arterial line read HR 102, NBP 83/55, MAP was 62 and O2 sat 100%. At 6:45 her MAP was 65, BP 92/59, HR 96 and O2 sat 99%.

At 7:00 her infectious disease doctor came in and informed me that her pathology report was back, and it showed that her pericardium had chronic inflammation. He said that she would need prophylactic therapy for the TB on an outpatient basis for the next 6 months. Her MAP was 68, BP 103/59, HR 103 and O2 sat 98%.

At 8:00 her MAP was 63, BP 85/56, HR 111 and O2 sat 98%. At 9 her MAP was 60, BP 90/51, HR 89 and O2 sat 98%. At 9:15 she was given Carafate 10 ml, sodium chloride nasal spray, magnesium oxide 400 mg tab and Mylicon 80 mg tab. At 10:00 she was given Carafate 10 ml, sodium chloride nasal spray, magnesium oxide 400 mg tab, and Indocin 50 mg/2 caps. She was also given tramadol 50 mg tab for a pain level of 4.

While writing this book, I noticed her nurse charted weakness and nausea for greater than 72 hours at 11:00. Her MAP was 65, BP 95/55, HR 80 and O2 sat 96%. The Tramadol was effective!

Her intake had been recorded as 1,969.9 ml's and output 4,650 ml's.

April 14 at 3:00 AM the arterial line read HR 84, NBP 96/62, MAP 70 and O2 sat 100%. She was given Zofran 2ml and Toradol 1 ml for a pain level of 5. At 3:30 the Zofran was not effective but the Toradol had brought her pain level down to a 2.

At 3:50 she was given Phenergan 1 ml. When her nurse gave her Phenergan, he gave it too fast and it caused Courtney's heart to react. She began having a hard time breathing and she started complaining of feeling funny and that the room was spinning. The tachycardic monitor began alarming. The charge nurse came in the room and I informed her that he pushed the Phenergan too fast causing Courtney to react.

While writing this book, I noticed in her medical records, her nurse charted nutrition was probably inadequate.

Her sodium was high again at 141.

At 6:00 the JP drain put out 20 ml's. At 6:45 her MAP was 54, BP 79/47, HR 93 and O2 sat 96%.

At 7:00 her cardiologist came in and reported 50 mL's from the JP drain in the last 24 hours. Courtney stated she was feeling better! She said she still had pain when inhaling but none at rest. She was still experiencing hypotension with systolic blood pressure in the low 90's and the Dopamine drip was down to 12 mcg. She was experiencing drowsiness and weakness, but she had a steady gait. He said so far, the effusion appears transudative, meaning fluid pressure in the blood vessels increases; and pressure exerted by blood proteins may also be decreased. These circumstances may cause fluid from the blood vessels to move into the pleural space. The pericarditis was viral. He stopped the Indocin and informed me that the metabolic acidosis had resolved! Praise God!

At 7:15 AM her MAP was 57, BP 86/49, HR 98 and O2 sat 97%. At 8:45 she was given Carafate 10 ml and her MAP was 68, BP 96/59,

HR 79 and O2 sat 100%. At 9:45 her MAP was 63, BP 97/55, HR 102 and O2 sat 99%.

At 10:00 she was given a multivitamin 1 tab, magnesium oxide 400 mg tab, Colchicine 0.6 mg tab, Toradol 1 ml for a chest pain level of 7, sodium chloride nasal spray, Zoloft 25 mg tab, MiraLAX 17 gm, Protonix 40 mg tab, and a suppository. Courtney and I agreed that she did not need the suppository. We felt that prune juice was the better choice. Therefore, her nurse gave her prune juice.

Her MAP was 61, BP 83/55, HR 101 and O2 sat 97%.

At 9:48 PT charted, "Pt c/o feeling "nauseated" toward end of tx and nsg present and aware. Pt left reclining in the recliner after tx with pt.'s mom and nsg present and was reclining in the recliner upon arrival eating breakfast. Pt presented with a slow gt pace and mod fatigued after tx. Pt cont. to seem really motivated to participate with PT at this time. Will continue with POC. Pt having chest pain with rating of 7. Nsg present and aware of pt.'s c/o pain after tx."

At 10:00 AM she was given Phenergan 1 ml. At 10:30 her MAP was 64, BP 89/57, HR 84 and O2 sat 95%.

At 11:00 she was complaining of constipation and nausea. She was experiencing drowsiness and weakness, but she had a steady gait. At 11:15 her MAP was 57, BP 81/49, HR 86 and O2 sat 97%. At 11:30 she was given Florinef which is a corticosteroid for treating postural hypotension. Her MAP was 61, BP 87/52, HR 83 and O2 sat 97%.

At noon, her MAP was 66, BP 91/57, HR 97 and O2 sat 100%. At 12:15 she was given Zofran 2 ml and Carafate 10 ml. At 12:30 her MAP was 57, BP 72/52, HR 102 and O2 sat 98%. At 12:45 the Zofran was effective, and her MAP was 62, BP 94/52, HR 101 and O2 sat 98%. At 1:45 her MAP was 70, BP 82/67, HR 106 and O2 sat 99%. I was getting scared again. I stood at the foot of her bed and prayed over her again.

At 2:43 OT charted," Pt seated in recliner with mother in room engaging in eating lunch. Pt treated for UE ex this pm to increase with ADLs/ADL transfer d/t decrease in strength. Pt performed 1 set/10 bil UE ex with red TheraBand in various planes and movements. Pt c/o min nausea and reported that lower abd "hurts a little with movement". Pt declined further tx at this time requesting to finish lunch and resume therapy in am.

This COTA concurred and pt. with no further needs. Will continue POC."

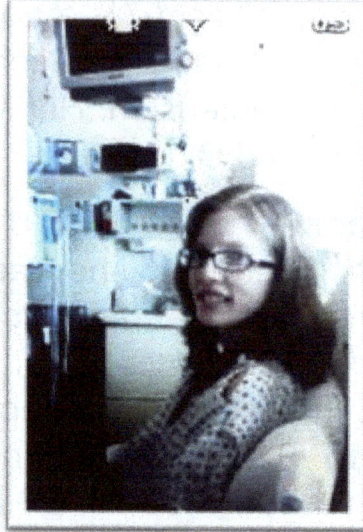

At 2:45 her MAP was 64, BP 86/58, HR 107 and O2 sat 98%.

At 3:00 PM her doctor came in and her nurse reported that she had turned the Dopamine drip down to 8 mcg. He informed me that Florinef, a corticosteroid, had been started. Courtney was complaining of some nasal stuffiness; therefore, Flonase had been ordered as well. Courtney's bowels had not moved since surgery and she was experiencing nausea. We had been complaining about this since her surgery on the 8th. Her nurse brought in a suppository. Courtney refused it and asked for prune juice instead. The JP drained out 10 ml's and her MAP was 56, BP 75/49, HR 109 and O2 sat 97%. She was experiencing some drowsiness and weakness, but she had a steady gait.

At 3:30 her MAP was 60, BP 88/53, HR 87 and O2 sat 98%. At 4:00 her MAP was 53, BP 82/45, HR 89 and O2 sat 98%. At 4:30 her MAP was 62, BP 90/54, HR 80 and O2 sat 97%. At 5:15 her MAP was 65, BP 94/57, HR 82 and O2 sat 97%. At 5:45 her MAP was 66, BP 102/56, HR 96 and O2 sat 99%. At 6:25 she was given Carafate 10 ml. At 8:00 her MAP was 79, BP 89/76, HR 111 and O2 sat 99%.

At 8:40 PM she was given Tylenol 650 mg/2 tabs, Carafate 10 ml, sodium chloride nasal spray, magnesium oxide 400 mg tab and Zofran 2 ml. Her MAP was 66, BP 98/58, HR 101 and O2 sat 98%. At 7:00 the Zofran was effective!

At 9:45 she was given Flonase 1 spray and the Tylenol was effective. At 10:00 her MAP was 69, BP 104/57, HR 84 and O2 sat 98%. At 10:15 she was given Mylanta 30 ml. At 10:45 her MAP was 58, BP 86/50, HR 89 and O2 sat 97%. At 11:00 her MAP was 64, BP 90/56, HR 88 and O2 sat 97%. At 11:15 her MAP was 63, BP 85/57, HR 101 and O2 sat 100%. At 11:30

her MAP was 66, BP 92/59, HR 83 and O2 sat 98%.

Her intake was recorded as 3,259 ml's and output 40 ml's with 8 urine counts.

April 15 at 12:30 AM she was given Mylicon 80 mg tabs and Tums 500 mg tabs. Her MAP was 65, BP 100/57, HR 98 and O2 sat 100%.

Her RBCs were even lower yet at 3.69, polychrome 1+, micro 1+, ovalocytes 1+ and plt clumps 1+. Hgb was even lower too at 11.1. Her anion gap was low but better at 7. BUN was low at 6 and BUN/Creat ratio was low at 10.

Polychrome is an abbreviation for polychromasia which is an abnormally high number of immature RBCs due to iron deficiency anemia. Polychromasia is a disorder that is a result of RBCs being prematurely released from the bone marrow during blood formation. Micro is abbreviated for microcytic anemia which is smaller than normal and decreased numbers of properly functioning RBCs which causes iron deficiency anemia. Ovalocytes, sometimes known as elliptocytes, are elongated or misshapen red blood cells. They are commonly seen in cases of iron-deficiency anemia. Platelet clumps are abnormal platelet clumping that can damage organs.

At 1:15 her MAP was 61, BP 88/53, HR 80 and O2 sat 97%. At 1:30 her MAP was 60, BP 95/49, HR 84 and O2 sat 99%. At 4:15 her MAP was 56, BP 80/48, HR 94 and O2 sat 96%. At 4:30 her MAP was 61, BP 86/52, HR 90 and O2 sat 97%. At 4:45 her MAP was 61, BP 92/52, HR 101 and O2 sat 98%.

At 5:00 the JP drain put out 30 ml's. At 5:45 her MAP was 52, BP 83/43, HR 95 and O2 sat 97%. At 6:45 her MAP was 64, BP 94/56, HR 109 and O2 sat 98%. At 7:00 the arterial line HR was 83, NBP 86/53, MAP was 61, HR 113 and O2 sat 97%. She was given Tylenol 650 mg/2 tabs. At 7:15 her MAP was 67, BP 95/58, HR 113 and O2 sat 96%.

At 7:30 AM her cardiologist came in and Courtney said she felt almost normal! She was up and walking again instead of lying in bed! Her bowels moved! The JP had drained 40 mL's in 24 hours. She had less nausea too! However, she was experiencing heartburn.

At 8:45 the Tylenol was effective, and her MAP was 60, BP 89/54, HR 102 and O2 sat 99%.

At 9:11 AM she was given a multivitamin 1 tab, magnesium oxide 400 mg tabs, Flonase nasal spray 1 spray, Florinef 0.1 mg tab, Colchicine 0.6 mg tab, Mylanta 30 ml, Carafate

10 ml, sodium chloride nasal spray, Zoloft 25 mg tab, MiraLAX 17 gm, and Protonix 40 mg tab.

At 9:30 her MAP was 65, BP 82/59, HR 114 and O2 sat 100%. At 10:15 her MAP was 62, BP 89/56, HR 115 and O2 sat 100%.

At 11:04 PT charted, "Performed AROM therapeutic exercises x30 reps ea. bil lower extremities sitting in the recliner after amb. AP, LAQ, MARCHES, ABD/ADD and PILLOW SQUEEZES. Pt left sitting in the recliner after tx with pt.'s mom present and was sitting in the recliner upon arrival. Pt amb without presenting with any unsteadiness/LOB, cont. to be motivated to progress and will D/C pt. from PT services at this time due to meeting all current goals and no further PT needed." This was an exciting yet disappointing day for Courtney. She was excited because she was done with PT, yet disappointed because she enjoyed PT and she got tired of sitting on her butt!

At 11:26 AM OT charted, "Pt seated in recliner with mother in room upon therapist arrival. Pt performed grooming ADLs completing oral hygiene with setup. Pt then donned bil socks. Pt declined LB dress at this time as pt. reported she is receiving sponge bath today and agrees to perform dressing this pm. Pt transfers on/off toilet without assistance. Pt performed bil UE ex with red TheraBand completing 2 sets/10 in all planes and movements with no c/o pain. Pt still demo weakness at bil UEs and would benefit from further ther ex for strengthening to increase with ADLs with pt. concurring. Pt seated in recliner after tx. Will f/u this pm for dressing ADLs and will continue POC."

At 12:15 it was charted that her nail beds were pale, she was a nutrition risk because she had been eating less than 50% of normal intake in the last 3 days. She had been experiencing nausea or heartburn for more than 72 hours.

At 12:30 PM she was given Carafate 10 ml and her MAP was 70, BP 85/66, HR 108 and O2 sat 100%. At 1:20 she was given Tylenol 650 mg/2 tabs. At 2:20 the Tylenol was effective. At 3:15 her MAP was 64, BP 89/56, HR 101 and O2 sat 99%.

At 3:20 OT charted, "Pt seated in recliner with mother in room upon therapist arrival. Pt performed dressing ADLs for LB dressing. Pt donned LB pants mod able to thread bil LEs into pants and stood from chair to complete dressing. Pt and mother reported pt. bathed self during sponge bath with assistance only for washing back. Pt transfers on/off toilet without assistance and performs self-cleaning. Pt performed bil UE ex with 2 lb. theraball in all planes and movements and took rest breaks between sets. Pt with no c/o pain throughout tx. Pt performs BADLs without assistance from helper and has met OT goals. Pt and mother both agree bil UE ther ex are beneficial to pt. at this time and requested to continue with OT tx for ex. Will continue POC with focus on preserving and increasing bil UE and endurance. Pt setting in chair after tx and call light near."

At 3:45 PM she was given Mylanta 30 ml. At 5:00 the JP drain put out 40 ml's and she was experiencing heartburn. She was given Carafate 10 ml. Her MAP was 63, BP 97/55, HR 86 and O2 sat 100%. At 6:45 her MAP was 74, HR 109, BP 88/69 and O2 sat 100%.

At 7:50 PM her arterial line HR was 115, NBP 102/70 and she was experiencing heartburn. At 8:00 she was given magnesium oxide 400 mg tabs and Carafate 10 ml. At 9:05 she was given sodium chloride nasal spray, Tylenol 650 mg/2 tabs and Flonase nasal spray.

At 10:05 the Tylenol was effective! At 10:15 she was given Mylanta 30 ml and Tums 500 mg tab.

At 11:45 her MAP was 66, BP 94/58 and O2 sat 98%.

Her intake was recorded as 3,974 ml's and her output 70 ml's with 10 urine counts.

April 16, at midnight she was experiencing heartburn. At 2:21 AM the nurse charted barriers to learning due to acuity of illness. At 4:00 she was tachycardic at 103, her MAP was 67, BP 88/61 and O2 sat 98%.

Her RBCs were even lower yet at 3.55, Hgb even lower at 10.6, Hct even lower at 31, monocytes low but better at 0.16, poik is 1+, and aniso 1+. Poik is abbreviated for poikilocytosis which is a blood disorder that causes abnormally shaped RBCs. The cause of poikilocytosis is a deficiency of vitamin B12 or folic acid. Aniso is abbreviated for anisocytosis which is unequal RBCs. Unequal RBCs is a sign of iron deficiency anemia.

At 5:45 she was given Tylenol 650mg/2 tabs.

Her weight was 99.6 pounds! She has gained 9 pounds! Her total gain was 16.6 pounds! Her nurse and I discussed how Courtney was gaining weight awfully fast. It was exciting but it was too fast! We both suspected that it was water weight from the IV fluid.

At 6:45 the Tylenol was effective! At 7:00 she had heartburn. At 9:25 she was given Flonase nasal spray, Florinef 0.1 mg tab, Colchicine 0.6 mg tab, sodium chloride nasal spray, Zoloft 25 mg tab, MiraLAX 17 gm, Protonix 40 mg tab, multivitamin 1 tab, magnesium oxide 400 mg tab and Carafate 10 ml.

At 11:40 OT charted, "Pt seated in recliner with mother in room upon therapist arrival. Pt performed bil UE ex with 2 lb. theraball in all planes and movements and took rest breaks between sets. Pt with no c/o pain throughout tx but did report soreness from ex yesterday stating, "It's a good kind of soreness." Will see pt. this pm to ed on HEP and issue TheraBand for pt. self ex as pt. is motivated to continue routine. Pt seated in chair after tx and call light near."

HEP stands for home exercise program.

At noon, her cardiologist came in. Courtney said she felt good! And she was walking around without difficulty! The JP drained 30 mL's in the last 24 hours. She had been taken off the Dopamine drip and she was stable to transfer to a regular room! Nasal congestion was her main complaint. She was taking Flonase nasal spray and saline nose spray, but one dose of Zyrtec (antihistamine) had been ordered. Naproxen had been discontinued.

At 12:45 PM she was given Zyrtec 10 mg tab and Carafate 10 ml.

At 2:42 her nurse charted barriers to learning due to acuity of illness.

At 2:50 PM OT charted, "Pt up amb with mother upon arrival. Pt amb down hall and back to room without assistance with no c/o pain. Pt d/c from ther OT tx d/t pt. performs BADLs without assistance and has met all goals. Pt received HEP and requires no further OT tx. Pt performed UE ex with yellow TheraBand in all planes and movements x1 set/10 per ex. Pt seated in chair with mother in room after tx and all questions answered." When Courtney found out she was being discharged from OT treatment, she cried. She cried because she was proud of what she had accomplished with therapy and how far she had come.

At 5:00 the JP drained out 35 ml's and she was given Mylanta 30 ml. At 5:30 she was given Carafate 10 ml.

At 6:00 her infectious disease doctor came in and informed us that the pericarditis was of unknown cause but not of pyogenic or mycobacterial cause per available information.

At 7:30 PM Courtney was transferred to a regular room!

Chapter 8

The Cardiac Floor

While writing this book, I noticed in Courtney's medical records, her nurse charted, "PO intake less than 50% of normal in last three days."

At 8:00 the Tylenol was effective! At 9:45 she was given sodium chloride nasal spray and Flonase nasal spray. At 10:00 she was given Carafate 10ml and magnesium oxide 400 mg tab. At 11:00 the nurse charted that Courtney had a barrier to learning due to acuity of illness.

Her intake was recorded as 2,210 ml's and output 95 ml's and 5 urine counts.

April 17 at midnight her MAP was 65, HR 47, BP 85/52, RR 18 and O2 sat 98%. At 2:00 AM the JP drained out 60 ml's. At 4:00 she was given Tylenol 650 mg/2 tabs for a pain level of 8.

She weighed 97.4 pounds. She had lost 2.2 pounds. Her BMI was 15.55.

At 5:00 AM the Tylenol was effective! At 7:00 her HR was 106, BP 80/52, and O2 sat 97%. At 8:20 she was given Flonase nasal spray, Florinef, Carafate 10 ml, sodium chloride nasal spray, Zoloft 25 mg tab, Protonix 40 mg tab, multivitamin 1 tab, and magnesium oxide 400 mg tab. Her HR was 105 and BP 95/58.

At 9:00 the order for the Colchicine was changed from daily to every other day. At 10:22 she had a pain level of 4. At 10:50 she was given Tylenol 650 mg/2 tabs for a pain level of 8.

At 11:00 the cardiologist came in and Courtney reported that her pain was being controlled with Tylenol! She had gained some weight too! He said her right and left ventricles were functioning properly! He stopped the IV fluid because it may have been what was contributing to the JP drain output.

Ya think!

At 11:50 the Tylenol was effective!

At 12:45 AM she was given Carafate 10 ml. At 6:15 she was given Carafate 10 ml. At 7:00 her MAP was 72, BP 85/66, RR 16 and O2 sat 98%.

At 8:30 the doctor came in and he informed me that he was still not happy with her blood pressure. He thought it was still too low. He ordered a complete blood count (CBC) and a comprehensive metabolic panel (CMP).

In the process of writing this book, I noticed that her nurse charted at 3:00 "Dx: Pericardial effusion s/p pericardial window, TB positive, hypotension, GERD. Nutrition Follow-Up Needed: Yes; Nutrition problem 1: involuntary weight loss; related to: unknown; evidenced by: recent 10# weight loss; status: ongoing; nourishments: yes; dietitian: yes."

At 9:00 she was given sodium chloride nasal spray, Flonase nasal spray, Mylicon 80 mg tab, Carafate 10 ml, and magnesium oxide 400 mg tab. At 10:20 she was given Tylenol 650 mg/2 tabs for a pain level of 4. At 11:20 the Tylenol was effective!

Her intake was recorded as 2,109 ml's and output 150 ml's with 9 urine counts.

April 18 at 12:30 AM Courtney was up walking the hall! She was complaining of gas on her stomach. She had been medicated. Her potassium and magnesium were low again. Her potassium was 3.4. Both had been replaced per protocol. Her RBCs were even lower at 3.17, RDW-CV was high at 16.4%, Hgb was lower at 9.6, Hct was lower at 29, eosinophil was high at 5.6, albumin was low at 2.9, total protein was even lower at 5.2, aspartate aminotransferase (AST) was high at 68.0, alanine aminotransferase (ALT) was high at 128.0, estimated creatinine clearance was 121.55

ml/min, eGFR African American was 185.31 and eGFR Non-African American was 152.90.

Eosinophils are a component of the immune system and can be elevated in patients with parasitic infections, fungal diseases, allergies, adrenal illnesses, skin disorders, toxin exposure, autoimmune disease, endocrine disorders and tumors. RDW-CV is red cell distribution width which is an indicator of iron deficiency anemia and folate deficiency.

Courtney had mild anemia.

An albumin blood test measures the amount of albumin in your blood. Albumin is a protein made by your liver. Albumin helps keep fluid in your bloodstream, so it does not leak into other tissues. It also carries various substances throughout your body, including hormones, vitamins, and enzymes. Low albumin levels can indicate a problem with your liver or kidneys.

I explained to him that Courtney had been struggling with anemia since she was a toddler.

AST and ALT are liver enzymes. Courtney's liver was struggling.

Creatinine is waste. Creatinine is filtered through the kidneys and excreted in urine. Doctors measure the blood creatinine as a test of kidney function. The kidneys' ability to handle creatinine is called the creatinine clearance, the rate of blood flow through the kidneys. GFR (glomerular filtration rate) is equal to the total of the filtration rates of the functioning nephrons in the kidney.

eGFR means the estimated GFR, because GFR cannot be measured directly. It is calculated based on two formulas. The calculation of GFR is based on a person's serum creatinine level and some variables including gender, age, weight and race.

Assume an American white and an African American have the same serum creatinine level, are at the same age and weight. In other words, there is a modification for African American in the calculation of GFR.

The modification is since African Americans have, on average, greater muscle mass and thus higher serum creatinine levels.

African American refers to the same reference chart.

When the GFR is calculated, both Caucasians and African Americans refer to the same reference table. The modification occurs only in the calculation.

Kidney damage:

Stage 1 – normal or minimal kidney damage with normal GFR, eGFR 90+

Stage 2 – mild decrease in GFR, eGFR 60-89

Stage 3 – moderate decrease in GFR, eGFR 30-59

Stage 4 – severe decrease in GFR, eGFR 15-29

Stage 5 – kidney failure, eGFR <15

For the age range of 20-29, the average estimated eGFR is 116.

Courtney's doctor ordered a celiac panel, ferritin level, hepatitis C antibody, vitamin B12 level and auto differential.

At 3:30 she weighed 97 pounds. She had lost 4 ounces.

At 4:30 she had a pain level of 6. At 7:15 she was given Tylenol 650 mg/2 tabs. At 8:00 she was given Protonix 40 mg tab, multivitamin 1 tab, magnesium oxide 400 mg tabs, Flonase nasal spray, Colchicine 0.6 mg tab, Carafate 10 ml, sodium chloride nasal spray, and Zoloft 25 mg tab.

At 8:15 the Tylenol was effective!

At 12:20 PM she was given Carafate 10 ml. At 1:30 she was given potassium chloride 20 meq orally. At 4:30 she was given Tylenol 650 mg/2 tabs for a pain level of 6 and Carafate 10 ml. At 6:30 the Tylenol was effective at lowering her pain level to a 2. At 7:00 her RR was 18,

HR 114, BP 113/54 and O2 sat 98%. At 8:50 she was given Flonase nasal spray, Carafate 10 ml, sodium chloride nasal spray, and magnesium oxide 400 mg tab. At 10:24 a nursing plan of care for self-care deficit, knowledge deficit, and anxiety was initiated.

At 10:56 PM she was given Tylenol 650 mg/2 tabs for a pain level of 6 and Mylanta 30 ml. At 11:56 the Tylenol had brought her pain level down to a 2.

Her intake was recorded as 200 ml's and output 40 ml's with 6 urine counts.

April 19, her total iron binding capacity (TIBC) was low at 248.4 and her transferrin was low at 166.7. The Hepatitis C test came back negative!

Transferrin is a protein produced by the liver. It regulates the absorption of iron into the blood. TIBC relates to the amount of transferrin in your blood that is available to attach to iron.

Although TIBC and transferrin are two different tests, they basically measure the same thing, so you will usually have either one or the other.

As transferrin is produced by the liver, the TIBC level will also be low if the person has liver disease.

At 7:00 she rated her pain at a 5.

At 7:30 AM her cardiologist came in and ordered to have the JP drain removed! She was given Tylenol 650 mg/2 tabs. At 8:15 she was given Carafate 10 ml, Zoloft 25 mg tab, Protonix 40 mg tab, multivitamin 1 tab, and magnesium oxide 400 mg tab.

At 8:30 the Tylenol had lowered her pain level to a 2. At 11:50 she was given Mylanta 30 ml.

At 1:50 PM she was given Carafate 10 ml and Zyrtec 10 mg tab.

At 2:15 her nurse came in to remove the JP drain and reported that all doctors had agreed to discharge her from the hospital!

Let's go home!

When she was discharged her potassium, magnesium and blood pressure were all still low. She was also still experiencing GERD.

The medications she was discharged with were:

Tylenol 325 mg/2 tabs every four hours

Mylanta 30 ml every four hours

Buspar 5 mg tab twice a day

Tums 500 mg tab every eight hours

Colchicine 0.6 mg every other day

Flonase nasal spray two times a day

Magnesium oxide 400 mg tabs twice daily

Protonix 40 mg tab daily

Sertraline 25 mg tab daily

MiraLAX 17 gm daily

Sodium chloride nasal spray 2 sprays twice a day

Carafate 10 ml 4 times a day

Multivitamin 1 tab daily

MiraLAX (daily)

Phenergan 25 mg tab every four hours as needed

Compazine (as needed)

Simethicone 80 mg tablet every six hours as needed

and one 20 meq dose of potassium.

Her doctor came in as discharge paperwork was being processed. He reminded me that some labs including celiac sprue panel and chronic anemia were still pending and to be sure and call later to get the results. He looked at her and he said, "She still doesn't look right. I still feel like there is something wrong that we are missing. I suspect an underlying malabsorption disorder associated with her weight loss. I know her cardiologist and surgeon have already discharged but I do not agree with discharge, so be careful. Symptomatically, she has much improved other than her severe acid reflux disease." I pray he reads this book.

Her discharge blood pressure was 93/59.

At 3:00 PM she was given Tramadol 50 mg tab for a pain level of 5. At 4:00 the Tramadol was effective! At 8:30 she was given Mylicon 80 mg tab, Mylanta 30 ml, and Carafate 10 ml.

We were given orders to follow up with her infectious disease doctor in 5-7 days, her cardiac surgeon in 3 weeks on May 10, 2015, her GI specialist in 1-2 weeks, her cardiologist in 2-4 weeks, and her primary physician in 5-7 days.

Chapter 9

Follow Up Appointments.

After discharge, her follow up visit with the cardiologist went great however, her stomach was still hurting.

May 1, 2015, I took Courtney to her PCP and she ordered an upper GI x-ray that revealed significant gastroesophageal reflux (GERD). She was also given a past medical history of unintentional weight loss, anxiety, palpitations, chronic constipation, and abnormal uterine bleeding.

May 8, 2015, I took Courtney to her GI specialist and he ordered a gastric emptying study which showed gastric emptying was delayed by 98 minutes. She was diagnosed with Gastroparesis.

Gastroparesis is a disorder that occurs when the stomach takes too long to empty food. This disorder leads to a variety of symptoms that can include nausea, vomiting, feeling easily full, and a slow emptying of the stomach, known as delayed gastric emptying. Gastroparesis can be due to a variety of issues.

What causes gastroparesis?

While the exact cause of gastroparesis is not known, it is thought to have something to do with disrupted nerve signals in the stomach. It is believed that when the nerves to the stomach become affected by a variety of factors, food can move through it too slowly.

May 20, 2015, she had an EGD. After her GI doctor performed the EGD he said that she was completely raw, and her stomach looked like raw hamburger meat. He proceeded to put her on antacids.

August 19, 2015, her GI specialist tested her for an autoimmune disorder. It came out negative. We do not have record of or remember which autoimmune disorder it was.

I texted several of my nursing friends asking what they suggested for acid reflux, since Courtney had tried everything over the counter, and nothing was working. One friend responded back and suggested baking soda. So, upon her suggestion, I mixed up one teaspoon of baking soda in about four ounces of water. It made Courtney vomit violently for the rest of the day, which consisted of four hours.

What I learned, when it comes to baking soda, if you consume anything that has baking soda (sodium bicarbonate) in it and it causes any stomach discomfort, then you have low stomach acid. If baking soda helps you experience stomach relief, then you have high stomach acid. Therefore, Courtney had low stomach acid.

A nursing friend that I graduated with told me about a holistic pharmacy here in Amarillo that could do a blood type test and tell what medications, food and supplements Courtney needed based on her blood type.

October 1, 2015, I started Courtney on his supplements including a refrigerated probiotic and she rode a health roller coaster and gained up to 100 pounds. She was taking ten different medications as well.

She was seeing a counselor because she was diagnosed with depression and anxiety while in the hospital. She was anticipating seeing a nutritionist as well.

October 8, 2015, we were nervous because she was seeing a new PCP. Courtney was still having severe abdominal pain, supposedly due to GERD. She was still complaining of indigestion despite using Dexilant, Cimetidine, Zantac, Gaviscon, Protonix and Tums (sometimes using multiple at one time). Since all these medications were not working, she was put on Reglan.

When she was in the hospital, she was diagnosed with latent TB (meaning she had been exposed). She was taking Isoniazid for the latent TB. Since she was seeing him for the first time, it was requested that I take all her medications and supplements in with us. He noticed the vitamin D and instructed me to take her off it. I asked him why. He said that if her level were elevated, she would have bad side effects. I asked him to check her level, he said it was not warranted. I told him I was going to keep her on it. He told me that if she suffered any consequences, it was all on me. I told him I would accept that responsibility.

October 28, 2015, I took her to her PCP for lab results. She was complaining of diarrhea and severe stomach pain that doubled her over. I took her off the Reglan because it was not working for her. Her PCP started her on Bentyl.

In October of 2015, I was introduced to Plexus supplements by a prior friend where I volunteered at. She recommended that since Courtney needed to gain weight, to start her on a protein shake. That made her sick.

Then, a Plexus supplement called Slim was recommended because Courtney was complaining of what she felt like was blood sugar issues. The Slim seemed to be helping some but she needed more. I found out about the Plexus probiotic called ProBio5. Within two weeks I saw a huge difference in her! This probiotic was what she needed! Oddly enough, I still was not completely convinced. However, I was spending less for Plexus supplements than what I was paying at that holistic pharmacy. The friend that introduced me to Plexus suggested that I talk with the pharmacist about Plexus supplements. I went back to the holistic pharmacy and asked the pharmacist if he had heard of Plexus. He said, without being able to make eye contact with me, "you're wasting your money".

However, I was seeing a much bigger and quicker difference in Courtney with the Plexus supplements than what I was seeing with his supplements. Although, I did keep her on his digestive enzyme called Robynzyme.

In October of 2015, her divorce was final!

In November of 2015, we both did our duty and went to Walgreens to get our flu shot.

December 1, 2015, her GI specialist ordered an upper GI with small bowel that showed mild GERD.

December 8, 2015, I took her back to her PCP. Courtney was complaining of a lot of gurgling, indigestion, and complaining that when she would eat it felt like the food was trying to go down, but something was fighting it. We informed her PCP that she was taking multiple homeopathies which seemed to be helping. However, we felt that the natural methods were fighting against the medications. Courtney and I felt strongly that the EGD needed to be repeated to make sure that the infection was cleared. Courtney was also experiencing a high heart rate (127) and at times she was feeling short of breath. Her potassium had gone down to 3.3, CO2 went down to 19, folate level was high at greater than 24.8 and vitamin B12 was deficient at 144.

The CO2, folate and vitamin B12 results were not revealed to me, however it all meant that she was becoming acidic, again. She was not methylating, and she was anemic. Her PCP ordered her to take potassium pills. I requested liquid since she was already dealing with stomach pain. Potassium pills are hard on the stomach.

December 16, 2015, her GI specialist refused to see Courtney and she was assigned to his NP. Courtney reported that she was feeling better. The diarrhea and abdominal bloating had resolved! However, she continued to struggle with gurgling and indigestion. She said she was eating better and eating a lot but not getting full. She was taking HCL and ProBio5. The NP informed us that Courtney's small bowel follow through was negative. I asked to see her test results which read that she had inflammation and slow digestion. I asked her, "You call that negative?" She recommended a psychiatric evaluation and diagnosed Courtney with irritable bowel. Courtney and I refused and walked out, never to go back again.

January 23, 2016, I was so impressed with Courtney's progress with the ProBio5, that I decided to join Plexus as an ambassador. If you decide that you want to give Plexus supplements a try, feel free to shop at this link mysite.plexusworldwide.com/kimseymour. My ambassador ID number is 1371269.

June 25, 2016, Courtney did a home spit test and unfortunately, due to her recently having to take pain medication and a muscle relaxer after our car wreck, the candida overgrowth had come back. However, she was already fighting back with Plexus supplements!

Have you ever heard of the candida overgrowth home spit test?

This is a simple test you can do at home!

Candida begins in the intestinal tract, where it sets up its ongoing production. As time goes by, the yeast migrates along the mucous membranes of the digestive tract into the stomach, then up the esophagus and finally into the mouth (sounds like GERD, right!). Often, depending on how thick the yeast becomes, it can be seen in the mouth and on the tongue as a white film called oral thrush. The fungal yeast mixes into the saliva and has certain properties (heavier than water) when put into water. Often, depending on how thick the yeast becomes, it can be seen in the mouth and on the tongue as a white film called oral thrush. The fungal yeast mixes into the saliva and has certain properties (heavier than water) when put into water.

When performing this simple test at home, be sure and use fresh bottled water, NOT tap water. Do this test first thing in the morning, before you brush your teeth, eat, or drink anything. Here is a link to further explain https://www.youtube.com/watch?v=Nb362iofKe k&fbclid=IwAR0GAL8UcMatnDS5LSXywOSEY Dfs6haO_nvSGwMfAm4K5kIhx9H73u8UiyE

Chapter 10

The Alternative Route

I took Courtney to an alternative NP and I was one relieved mom! Her new alternative NP's exact words were, "EVERYTHING STEMS FROM THE GUT. You CAN NOT get all the nutrition your body needs from food alone. It is impossible. You have to have supplements."

When I told Courtney's alternative NP about the western medicine doctors giving up and recommending a psychiatric evaluation, we got the look of compassion I was hoping for! Courtney ate Hippocrates soup for a while. Courtney's NP said the most important thing for her to drink was bone broth. She put her on a different and less harsh digestive enzyme and ordered lab work. She knew about candida overgrowth and she said that sometimes she orders for her patients to do a home spit test! She gave Plexus supplements two thumbs up!!!!! However, she said that Courtney simply needed more supplements. She did not suspect any organ damage; however, she did think that Courtney's adrenals and thyroid were out of balance. She said that she never recommends over the counter supplements, because even they are still too harsh.

May 30, 2017, Courtney was put on Gastrozyme, 2 capsules with meals. It was suggested to make Hippocrates soup and to make homemade chicken bone broth using an organic chicken. Courtney's NP also ordered a home saliva test to check her hormones.

Her lab results were as follows: "Vitamin C level is very good. fasting glucose is good at 88. Fasting insulin is a little elevated at 6.57. Optimal is 5. Ferritin is on the low side at 32. Optimal is 100. Folate is high at greater than 26.40. Thyroid: No auto-immune thyroid disease. TSH is high at 4.39, optimal is 1. Free T4 is good at 1.19. Free T3 is good at 3.64. Magnesium is good at 2.2. Phosphorus is low at 2.8. Uric acid is great. B12 is high at 1037 indicating liver inflammation. Vitamin D is low at 32. Chronic Epstein Barr Virus titer is positive and white blood cells are low at 4.6 indicating a virus is active and her immunity is low. That virus is Chronic Epstein Barr Virus (CEBV). CO_2 is low at 21.0 (but it is better! Remember in the hospital it was 20.0?) and anion gap is high at 17.9." (Emphasis added) Remember in the hospital it was low at 6?

The anion gap tells you how much acid is in your blood. Too much acid in the blood can be a sign of short-term problems like dehydration and diarrhea.

I told Courtney's NP that it was impossible for her to be dehydrated because she drinks half her body weight in ounces of water a day. She asked, "Then how much salt does she eat with her food?" I said, "I don't cook with salt." She told Courtney to add a pinch of sea salt to every glass of water per day. So, now that the fluid had been taken off her heart, her anion gap was high.

June 9, I finally figured out how to make homemade chicken bone broth!

Would you like to know how to make my homemade chicken bone broth?

I buy a whole organic chicken, wash it and put it in a crock pot for 7 hours with Kangen water. After it is thoroughly cooked, I debone it also removing skin, fat, most of the meat and cartilage.

Put the bones, skin, fat, cartilage, and some meat in an Instant Pot with chicken feet. Cook for 4 hours. When you can stab through the bone with a fork, it is done.

Strain the broth from the bones. Be sure to double strain so you do not get any bone fragments in your broth.

Enjoy!

Store in fridge overnight. It will gel in the fridge.

June 14, 2017, we got Courtney's lab results. Her NP charted, "Vitamin C level is very good. Fasting glucose was good at 88. Fasting insulin is a little elevated at 6.57. Optimal is 5. Ferritin is on the low side at 32. Optimal is 100. Folic acid is perfect. Thyroid: No auto-immune thyroid disease. TSH is high at 4.39, optimal is 1. Free T4 is good at 1.19. Free T3 is good at 3.64. Magnesium is good at 2.2. Phosphorus is low at 2.8. Uric acid is great. B12 is good. Vitamin D is low at 32.

Foods: A level of < 2 is normal, 15 is high and 30 is very high. Cow's milk protein antibody is 50.5, corn 10.5, oats 7.3, eggs (yolk and white) 7, wheat 6.8, soybean 4.1 and peanuts 4." Her food allergy testing was done via blood.

Do you remember the protein shake from Plexus supplements that made Courtney sick? It had milk in it! That is why it made her sick.

Courtney was taking Plexus ProBio5 (probiotic), Plexus MegaX (omegas) 2 gel caps daily, Plexus Slim daily, Plexus VitalBiome (probiotic, 30 to 40 billion good bacteria), Plexus XFactor Plus 2 capsules daily, Cell

Ready Minerals 1 ounce twice daily, Vitamin D3 2000 u/drop take 25 drops under tongue x3 days and then take 5 drops under tongue daily, and Gastrozyme 2 capsules with each meal (may take as needed for heartburn or nausea).

It was suggested that Courtney try to decrease her meat intake and increase her vegetable intake. Courtney hated doing this because she did not get full.

June 20, I made Hippocrates soup. Hippocrates soup ingredients are red onion, red potato, leek, garlic and celery.

July 6, 2017, Courtney's NP charted, "Estradiol level is good. Progesterone level is very low. You do not have enough progesterone to balance your estrogen. DHEA is low. Testosterone is low.

Adrenals: Your cortisol level is high in the morning, at lunch and at supper. Your cortisol level is low at bedtime."

DHEA is made in the brain. It is a natural steroid hormone. It is the "mother hormone". It is the source that fuels the body's metabolic pathway.

Cortisol helps the body use sugar (glucose) and fat for energy (metabolism) and manage stress. It is a steroid hormone. It is responsible for immune responses, metabolism, and anti-inflammatory.

Supplements she was taking: Plexus ProBio5, Plexus XFactor Plus, Plexus MegaX, Adrenal Support Plus Capsules take 1 capsule in the morning, Cortisol High Potency Liquid take 3 drops under tongue in the morning and at lunch, Vitamin D3 2000 u/drop take 5 drops under tongue daily, PaxImmune 2 sprays under tongue twice daily, and Progensa Mist apply 1 spray topically daily.

It was recommended that Courtney take 4 Digestzyme and 1 HCL Plus when she eats vegetables. Take 1 HCL Plus when she eats meat only.

To overcome an allergy, it takes two years for every two points if you leave the offending allergen completely alone. Therefore, Courtney will be 50 years old when she overcomes her cow's milk allergy. In eight years, she will overcome her peanut allergy, 2x4=8.

July 31, Courtney's NP took her off solid veggies and put her back on Hippocrates soup until more food allergy testing is done. If you are not digesting food properly, you could be allergic to it. Do not push your body to do something it is telling you "no" to. Courtney had been taking Plexus supplements for 2 years at this point and according to her N.P., they saved her life! However, since she was still so sick, she simply needs more supplements than what

Plexus offers currently (which we buy from the doctor's office, not from over the counter).

We also needed to add in nutrition. This was the main reason I wanted to bring Courtney to this doctor's office. I needed to learn more about nutrition, and I needed to learn it fast.

As per her NP, Courtney needed 10,000 units daily of vitamin D3 and 30 to 40 billion good bacteria. Her NP did not put her on an iron supplement because it would have been too hard on her stomach. We used nutrition to get her iron up. She also did not want to put her on any medication for her thyroid because she did not feel it was low enough for medication and over time nutrition will balance that out.

Courtney had also been taken off the Plexus VitalBiome because it contains milk. So, why is dairy such a problem? Have you heard of Leaky Gut?

The arrangement between yeast and your body has been broken. The fungus has learned how to attack and enter your body. It sinks its tentacles deep into your tissue, and when it hits your bloodstream, it goes crazy. Once it has a taste of your blood, it wants more and more and more, and it goes on a wild feeding frenzy.

Your bloodstream is the "highway" to every cell in your body. Infiltration into your bloodstream is the turning point for your immune system. All your organs and glands, all your tissues are exposed.

Now fungus has access to your entire body, and it wants everything it sees.

With the fungi's new tentacles, the once peaceful parasite can poke holes through all the mucosal linings of your body, especially your digestive tract, on its way to your blood.

Once your immune systems defense has been penetrated by fungus, your lining is punctured and weakened by its fungal tentacles. Fungal spores and their poisons enter through the holes into your bloodstream and start spreading to cells and organs. Immediately they start to disarm and depress your immune system. Some even reach your brain!

And so, a new disease has been born, called "leaky gut syndrome ".

August 8, 2017 her vitamin D was high at 147.03, white blood cell (WBC) was lower at 3.7, red blood cell (RBC) was high at 5.58, hemoglobin was high at 16.5 and hematocrit was high at 49.5.

Courtney has overcome the anemia by eating spinach daily!

August 14, 2017, I had been doing research on how our home environment affects our health. And, after reading *Recaging the Beast*, I knew about Thieves household cleaner. I had also been experimenting with Young Living essential oils. After talking with Courtney's NP about Young Living essential oils, I decided to become a distributor. If you decide that this is an option for you as well, feel free to shop here https://www.youngliving.com. My ID number is 12668940.

August 16, her NP charted, "Fasting glucose is 70. Insulin is 3.29, which is very good. Kidneys are good (remember two years ago, her kidneys were shutting down?), liver is good. Magnesium and phosphorus (she was on a supplement 6 weeks ago) is good. Thyroid is better. TSH is 3.4. This has improved from 4.39. Vitamin D is 147. This should be 75 to 100. We are going to cut back on her vitamin D dose." (Emphasis added)

Instead of doing food allergy testing via blood test to see what vegetables she can tolerate, we opted for a less invasive and less expensive test, muscle testing. We tested only a few vegetables and decided to test more later.

We found out she was allergic to leeks and garlic, which were two ingredients of Hippocrates soup. However, her body liked spinach, carrots and avocado. So, she started with avocado!

After doing the ART testing we eliminated some of the supplements that she was on and added a few. I was flabbergasted by this test! One of the new supplements was edible clay (Diatomaceous Earth) which is good for gut healing.

If you want to know more about ART testing (muscle testing) you can go to https://www.youtube.com/watch?v=5bK3ol5ZkH 0&fbclid=IwAR27xGrSTW5tBBqTo1hrkD3VFffV E82Q4rgn-4rxlG2l67dkvsHzF06K1il

This is the best and easiest to understand video I could find about Muscle Testing (ART) or Autonomic Response Testing. This can be done to detect foods and supplements that are best for you; what vaccines you have an injury to; what heavy metals you are sensitive to; etc.

The bitter-sweet news was the Chronic Epstein Barr Virus labs were better but her white blood cell count was extremely low, lower than it was. This meant her immunity was extremely low. We started her on Vitamin C intravenously (IV). She went two times per week for eight weeks.

She was taking Plexus ProBio5, Plexus XFactor Plus Multivitamin 2 capsules daily, Diatomaceous Earth one teaspoon mixed with water and drink daily, Adrenal Support Plus Capsules one capsule daily in the morning, Cortisol High Potency Liquid 3 drops under tongue in the morning and at lunch, Guna Liver 5 pellets melted under tongue before meals, Vitamin D3 2000 u/drop 2 drops under tongue daily in the morning, Probiotic 42.5 one capsule daily (sometimes 2 probiotics are needed), PaxImmune 2 sprays under tongue twice daily, and Progensa Mist 1 spray topically daily, increase to 3 sprays on days 12 to 26.

It was recommended to take the onion out of the Hippocrates soup simply because it was bothering Courtney's stomach. Decrease vitamin D3 to 2 drops every morning. Start 1 teaspoon of Diatomaceous Earth mixed in water daily and deep breathing daily. For the deep breathing she was supposed to inhale slowly counting to 8; hold for count of 8; exhale slowly with pursed lips. Take 10 breaths.

August 21, Courtney had her second vitamin C IV. It was called Myer's Cocktail with homeopathic sips. It was a combination of ascorbic acid, methylated B12, B complex vitamins, engystol, folic acid, lactated ringers, magnesium chloride, nux vomica-homaccord and trace minerals. The infusion took an hour. The only sign of candida die-off she had was a little acne. For the most part, she was having more energy and becoming more independent! The treatment made her hungry and thirsty though.

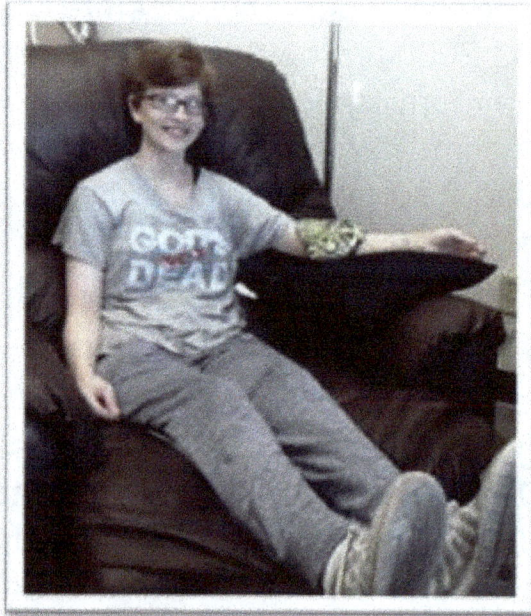

What is candida die-off?

Any time you start a probiotic or a prebiotic there is a chance that your body will experience something called candida die-off...which is the nasty TOXINS leaving your body! It is a good thing, but it may not feel good for a little while. Education is KEY & it is important.

When yeast and fungal cells are rapidly killed, a die-off occurs, and metabolic by-products (their poop) is released into your body. The amount of Candida cells being killed makes this quite different from your regular cell elimination. When these cells die, they release all the noxious substances that they contain.

This includes ethanol, uric acid, and acetaldehyde.

Acetaldehyde, is a known neurotoxin, which has a whole host of detrimental effects on your health and wellbeing. It can impair your brain function and even kill brain cells. Your endocrine, immune and respiratory systems can all be affected. It also damages the membranes of your red blood cells (RBCs), reducing their ability to carry oxygen throughout your body. You can see how excess acetaldehyde can quickly contribute to non-specific symptoms like brain fog and fatigue. These noxious by-products also cause allergic reactions and inflammation that lead to an array of undesirable symptoms.

Candida die-off symptoms will vary from

person to person, as each will have different degrees and types of infestation. If you are having severe die-off symptoms, there is one important thing that you can do, slow down your treatment and reduce your dosage. The liver is your main pathway for eliminating toxins, and the die-off symptoms mean that it is being overwhelmed.

What are candida die-off symptoms?

The symptoms of candida die-off are sometimes compared to those of a common cold or seasonal allergy but can be quite different from person to person. The toxic byproducts of candida overgrowth tend to cause inflammation, which can lead to a stuffy nose, blocked sinuses, and other allergy-type symptoms. Metabolites like the neurotoxin acetaldehyde can also cause symptoms like brain fog, headaches, fatigue, and nausea. Remember that these toxins are stressing your liver too, so having a sore abdomen (especially in the liver region) is also possible.

HERE ARE SOME DIE-OFF SYMPTOMS: Make sure you are drinking lots of water to flush out your system!!!

Headache, fatigue, dizziness

Swollen glands
Bloating, gas, constipation or diarrhea
Increased joint or muscle pain
Elevated heart rate
Chills, cold feeling in your extremities
Body itchiness, hives or rashes
Sweating
Fever
Skin breakouts

August 25, Courtney had another Myer's Cocktail IV infusion.

August 28, her 4th Myer's Cocktail. For 3 days she had been getting herself ready for the day and she was back to taking care of her dog!

September 1, another Myer's Cocktail. It was a mixture of ascorbic acid, methylated B12, B complex, folic acid, lactated ringers, magnesium chloride and trace minerals. The nurse did not put the engystol and nux vomica-homaccord in it.

September 6, another Myer's Cocktail. No engystol but the nux vomica-homaccord was added.

September 8, her 7th Myer's Cocktail (Vitamin C) treatment. She was able to get herself ready for the day without taking any breaks! She had been walking around more than sitting down. She had so much more energy, however she had to pace herself. Her brain fog had lifted! I was having to reteach her some cognitive things since she had the brain fog for so long. She was making excellent progress!

September 11, more Myer's Cocktail for immune support. Again, no engystol. Her 8th Myer's Cocktail (Vitamin C) treatment. Her cognitive process had already improved! She was able to help around the house again!

Engystol is homeopathic. It is for stimulation of the immune system in viral infections.

Nux vomica-Homaccord is a homeopathic used to treat a variety of diseases and functional disorders of the gastrointestinal (GI) tract.

Indications for this remedy:

- Liver tonic
- Aids digestion.
- Treatment of mild digestive disorders.
- Assists detoxification
- Male infertility and impotence
- Colds and flus, particularly in the early stages of the virus
- Allergies

- Back pain
- Irritability, impatience, and high sensitivity to stimuli, caused by stress or mental strain
- Headaches and migraine symptoms such as a sore scalp, frontal lobe pain, light sensitivity, or stomach problems
- Menstrual problems
- Insomnia

Nux Vomica Homaccord stimulates the gastrointestinal (GI) tract excretion pathway as well as the hepatic (liver) system. It has anti-inflammatory properties and contains powerful antioxidants. The flowers of nux vomica-homaccord also have antibacterial properties. These properties could potentially be beneficial for use in antiseptics.

September 13, 2017 her blood urea nitrogen (BUN) was high at 28, red cell distribution width (RDW) was high at 15.5.

High BUN levels are usually caused by a problem with your kidneys. Kidney damage can lead to a variety of symptoms, including weakness, shortness of breath, confusion, and fatigue. High BUN levels can also be caused by dehydration, stress, burn injuries, or gastrointestinal (GI) bleeding.

The RDW is the measurement in size and volume variations of the red blood cells (RBC).

Mostly, your doctor may request an RDW blood test under suspicion of the following situations:

- Anemia
- Cancer
- Cardiovascular Diseases
- Liver Diseases
- Any blood disorders

Courtney had a nutrient deficiency and we needed to reduce the inflammation in her liver.

We tested Courtney for Epstein Barr Virus. On her ANA screen with reflex to titer and pattern, it was positive. ANA pattern was homogeneous, and titer shows low antibody level at 1:640. Her DNA (da) antibody was negative at less than 1. However, her complement component C3c and C4c were low. C3c was 82 and C4c was 15.

These results were NOT presented to me by her alternative NP. I knew that her ANA was being tested because I was given the order to take to the lab. I had no idea what an ANA was, so I looked it up. I kept seeing the word autoimmune and I got nervous. I then thought, ok, no need to dwell on this. I will just wait and see what the result is.

When we went back to her NP for the results, she asked me! She said, "I'm sure that you saw that I wrote an order for an ANA and I'm sure that you looked it up." I said, "Yes." She told us that Courtney had Chronic Epstein Barr Virus (CEBV). I knew that I saw autoimmune and that CEBV was autoimmune. However, she was not sure about the ANA. She said she was going to have to talk with the doctor and show him her records and labs and get back with me on what he said.

The next day, she called and told me that we had tested for ESR which is an inflammatory marker and ANA which is a titer for autoimmune diseases. Her sed rate from the ESR was 6 indicating no inflammation. However, her ANA was positive and indicating a low antibody level. This caused us to wonder if she had lupus, another autoimmune disease. After talking with the doctor, he said that it just meant she had a little inflammation.

However, while writing this book, looking over her lab work and doing research, it seems to me that she indeed did have lupus.

Please allow me to explain, based on her lab results and her signs and symptoms (as many internet resources tell you to do), it seems to me that she had subacute cutaneous lupus erythematosus.

Today is September 25, 2020, she still has these rashes. They never bother her. To this day she has a discoid rash on her right wrist and a subacute cutaneous lupus erythematosus rash on the back of each arm. Her right arm is worse than the left.

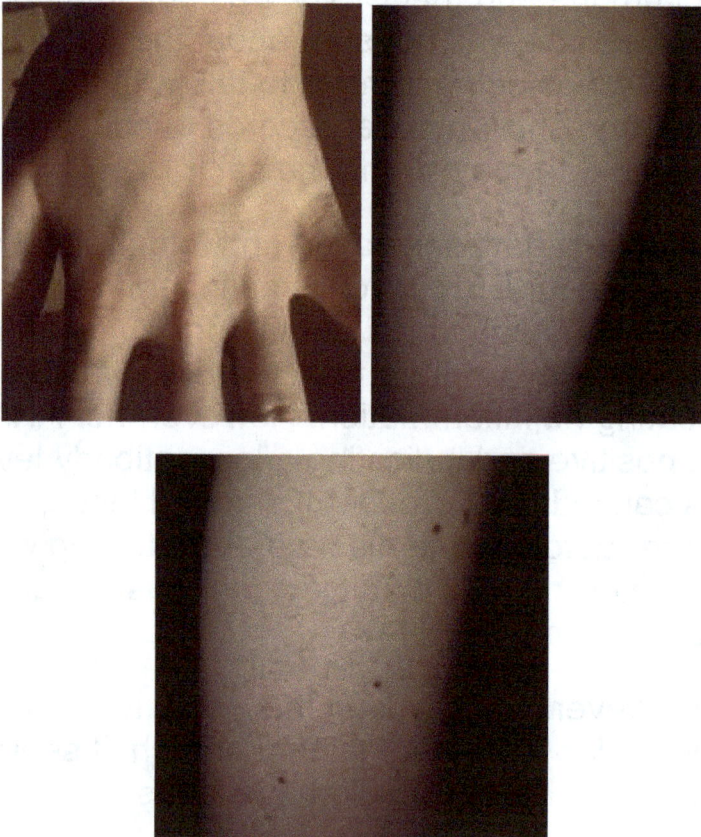

I am going to explain her labs for lupus and let you know what her signs and symptoms were. Feel free to get in touch and give me your thoughts, Courtney and I would love to hear from you.

ANA means autoimmune antinuclear antibodies. This literally means 'substance against the cell nucleus'. The nucleus is the 'headquarters' of the living cell; therefore, the ANA can damage or destroy cells & tissues.

95%-98% of patients with SLE will have a positive ANA test, however most people with a positive ANA test do not have SLE. A positive ANA test can be found in many conditions.

Antinuclear is a protein in the nucleus of a cell. Antibodies are made by WBCs, more specifically, the B lymph. IFA is indirect immunofluorescence antibody, that was positive. ANA pattern was homogeneous and ANA titer was 1:640.

The titer shows how many times the technician had to mix fluid from Courtney's blood to get a sample free of ANAs. Thus, a titer of 1:640 shows a greater concentration of ANA than 1:320 or 1:160, since it took 640 dilutions of the plasma before ANA was no longer detected. In fact, the difference between titers of 1:160 & 1:320 is only a single dilution. This means it was diluted 3 times before it was no longer seen. Which means a low antibody level. This is mostly seen in elderly people!

She was 25 years old when this test was done!

The homogeneous (diffuse) pattern is the most common pattern seen. The entire nucleus of the cell is seen. This pattern is usual in lupus. Even though her kidneys have been involved in the past, during her hospital stay, the DNA (ds) Antibody was negative at less than 1. Indicating she is negative for kidney lupus.

The complement system is a series of more than 15 proteins that assemble in domino fashion to destroy bacteria and viruses invading the body. The signal that initiates the domino cascade (called "activating" complement) is that an antibody meets an antigen (the bacterium or virus). Because lupus autoantibodies give the same signal and activate complement, the measurement of complement can be used to monitor lupus.

Because they give sufficient information, it usually suffices to measure only two of the complement proteins, called C3 and C4. Complement Component C3c being low indicates that she was prone to infection. And she had an active viral or bacterial infection. Complement Component C4c is low at 15 indicating viral or bacterial infection, inflammation in her liver, malnutrition and lupus.

A positive ANA test does not mean that a person has Lupus. The physician needs to find other clinical features such as rashes, arthritis, pleurisy, blood abnormalities, kidney disease, etc., in addition to a positive ANA test before making a diagnosis of SLE. A diagnosis of lupus is based on symptoms, physical examination abnormalities, and laboratory tests.

Not all patients with SLE have anti-dsDNA. Her signs and symptoms that have matched for years are inflammation, arthritis (possibly rheumatoid arthritis (RA)), discoid rash, heat rash (she got these frequently as a child during the summer), oral ulcers, acidosis, anemia, weight loss, electrolyte imbalance, leukopenia (low WBCs) and pericardial effusion.

Subacute cutaneous lupus erythematosus (SCLE) is characterized by the presence of nonscarring, photosensitive lesions that can take one of two distinct forms: (1) papulosquamous lesions that resemble psoriasis, or (2) annular-polycyclic lesions with peripheral scale and central clearing. These two forms can occur concurrently. SCLE has a predilection for the back, neck, shoulders, and extensor surfaces of the arms and usually spares the face. Courtney's rashes are on the extensor surfaces of her arms and the back of her hand, as shown in the pictures above.

The most common presenting manifestations are constitutional symptoms (fatigue and/or weight loss), cutaneous manifestations (e.g., rash), and articular manifestations (arthritis). Each of these manifestations appears to be present in at least 50% of lupus patients at the time of diagnosis. The other clinical features of SLE are much less likely to be presenting manifestations, although virtually any of them might be the first clue to the correct diagnosis.

September 15, 2017, her 9th Myer's Cocktail with ascorbic acid, methylated B12, B complex, folic acid, lactated ringers, magnesium chloride, nux vomica-homaccord, and trace minerals. Her nurse said she was starting to have a glow to her and a twinkle in her eye! I had not noticed since I am with her 24/7. That was so good to hear!

September 18, her 10th Myer's Cocktail (Vitamin C) treatment. At the beginning of this summer, 2017, she could not walk without assistance. At this point, she was not only walking on her own, but she was getting herself ready for the day and able to help around the house!

September 22, her 11th Myer's Cocktail (Vitamin C) treatment.

September 27, her NP charted, "CBC looks good. White count is 6.8. Red blood cells look good. Magnesium and phosphorus are perfect. LDH and ESR are good. ANA is positive. This means you have auto-immune disease."

The supplements Courtney was taking were: Plexus ProBio5, Plexus XFactor Multivitamin 2 capsules daily, Diatomaceous Earth one teaspoon mixed with water and drink daily, Adrenal Support Plus Capsules one capsule daily in the morning, Cortisol High Potency Liquid 3 drops under the tongue in the morning and at lunch, Guna Liver 5 pellets melted under tongue before meals, vitamin D3 2000 u/drop take 2 drops under tongue daily, Probiotic 42.5 one capsule daily, PaxImmune 2 sprays under tongue twice daily, and Progensa Mist 1 spray topically daily, increase to 3 sprays on days 12 to 26. She also had a Myer's Cocktail infusion.

It was recommended to continue the IV infusions. However, we are given the option of going to once a week, instead of twice a week. Courtney was experiencing what we call "gurgling" with her menstrual cycles. Therefore, we increased the Diatomaceous Earth to 1.5 teaspoons with her cycles. We decided to slowly add in one food at a time and see how she tolerates them. We were going to start going for walks in the neighborhood.

September 29, we decided to keep the Myer's Cocktail (Vitamin C) infusions going for a little while longer. We wanted to keep her immunity up during the "flu season" and the infusions were helping so much with her energy! She was no longer having symptoms of candida die-off! We were looking forward to a more active lifestyle!

October 3, another Myer's Cocktail infusion.

October 6, with Courtney nearing the end of her Myer's Cocktail (Vitamin C) infusions, I had observed that the explosion of yeast and yeast-related illnesses was trying to teach us an important lesson of survival. Like all hard lessons, if we learn from our mistakes and use what we have learned for the good, then the experience of having been ill and then overcoming the illness, will have been put to good use. Because God never takes us through storms without a reason.

If we see yeast infection as a "wake-up call," and take the warning seriously, we may have time to regroup and rebuild our defenses. In the end, we might even thank them for waking us up to our errors and giving us a chance to correct them.

By alerting us to our weaknesses, yeast is giving us a second chance. If we can "clean up our act," do a thorough house-cleaning and "throw out the trash", we may have time to turn the brewing candida overgrowth calamity around. If not, the acceleration of yeast overgrowths can become irreversible, as will be our early death.

We pray that you will be empowered to back the rampaging beast back into its cage and establish peace again. Living in harmony with wholeness of spirit, mind, and body, we can become free to become our optimal selves.

Perhaps candida overgrowth has come to expose us to ourselves. It is giving us both a challenge to grow and learn and an opportunity to transform ourselves more in His image, clean and full of light.

October 9, another Myer's Cocktail infusion.

October 14, we took a road trip and Courtney did NOT experience any motion sickness! Exactly five months ago, we took a road trip, and she came back home sick. Now, we are back in church! This is the active lifestyle we have been waiting for!

October 19, Myer's Cocktail (Vitamin C) IV treatment.

October 22, 2017, after seeing a Kangen water system in Courtney's NP's office waiting room, I decided to purchase a K8 water system and become an affiliate. If you decide you are interested in a Kangen water system, feel free to order from here: https://www.enagic.com. My sponsor ID number is 7322664 and my email is kim.seymore@sbcglobal.net. Please do not be concerned about the misspelling of my last name. Even when I spelled it correctly for AT&T, they still spelled it wrong!

October 26, this Myer's Cocktail infusion contained engystol.

November 15, Courtney was taking: Plexus ProBio5, Plexus MegaX (omegas) 2 gel caps daily, Plexus XFactor Plus Multivitamin 2 capsules daily, Diatomaceous Earth 1 teaspoon mixed with water and drink daily, Adrenal Support Plus Capsules 1 capsule daily in the morning, Cortisol High Potency Liquid 3 drops under tongue in the morning and at lunch, Guna Liver 5 pellets melted under tongue before meals, vitamin D3 2000 u/drop 2 drops under tongue in the morning, Probiotic 42.5 take 1 capsule daily, PaxImmune 2 sprays under tongue twice daily, and Progensa Mist 3 sprays topically daily, increase to 6 sprays on days 12 to 26. She had a Myer's Cocktail infusion today with engystol. She was complaining of having extremely uncomfortable gas. It was recommended that she start Eubioflor 5 drops 3 times daily.

November 29, 2017 her BUN was high at 22. This was better than it was in September! Her vitamin B12 was high at greater than 1500, folate was high at greater than 26.40, and WBCs low at 3.4.

November 30, 2017 her lab work was positive for Epstein-Barr Virus. EBV VCA AB (IGG) was high at 609.00 and EBV EBNA AB (IGG) was high at 292.00. These labs indicate a past infection meaning Chronic Epstein Barr Virus (CEBV). Her vitamin A was low at 31.

Chapter 11

Vaccine Injuries Revealed

December 15, 2017, Courtney took another home hormone saliva test. We got the results back December 22nd and it showed that she was pre-menopausal! She was still menstruating, and her last menses was 11/24/17. She was 26 years old and her BMI was 17.7, height 5 feet 4 inches, weight 103 pounds and her waist was 29 inches. Her ratio:pg/e2 was low at 52, estradiol low at 0.6 (premenopausal), progesterone was low at 75, testosterone low at 13, DHEAS low at 1.6 and her noon cortisol was high at 6.6.

She was put on topical progesterone spray, twice daily sublingual (under the tongue) cortisol, sublingual vitamin D3 and magnesium.

December 18, Courtney had Flu A+. Her NP put her on vitamin D3 50,000 units for 3 days and then decrease dose to 4,000 units daily. Vitamin C twice daily. A homeopathic for viruses of which she was to take 5 drops twice daily. Chamomile tea steam inhalations for her lungs. Her NP said if she was not better in a few days then we needed to consider a vitamin C IV treatment.

January 2, 2018, Courtney's NP charted, "CBC: WBC is low at 3400. Vitamin A is low at 31. Vitamin D is good at 66. B12 and folic acid are good. Thyroid could be better. Estradiol is low. Progesterone is low. Testosterone is low. DHEA is low. Adrenals are better."

Supplements Courtney was taking: Nature-Throid (this is actually a medication) 32.5 mg take one tablet in the morning on an empty stomach with a glass of water, Plexus ProBio5, Diatomaceous Earth one teaspoon mixed with water and drink daily, Ther-Biotic one capsule daily, Plexus MegaX (omegas) two gel caps daily, Plexus XFactor Multivitamin two capsules daily, Adrenal Support Plus one capsule daily in the morning, Guna Liver five pellets before meals, Vitamin D3 2000 u/drop two drops under tongue in the morning, Bio-Ae-Mulsion Forte (vitamin A) ten drops under tongue daily x3 days and then take 2 drops under tongue daily, PaxImmune 2 sprays under tongue twice daily, and Progensa Mist 3 sprays topically daily, increase to 6 sprays topically days 12 to 26.

Recommendations were: "Bio-adaptogen 1 capsule daily. Stop cortisol H drops. Vitamin A 10 drops daily x3 days and then take 2 drops daily. With Nature-Throid, wait 45 minutes before eating or taking other supplements. Peppermint tea or marshmallow root tea to combat nausea caused by Nature-Throid. Stop Eubioflor. Change to Therbiotic when you are finished with Probiotic 42.5. Start a gratitude journal and every night write 3 things that you are grateful for."

Her cortisol levels were normal! She no longer needed a cortisol supplement! Her Chronic Epstein Barr Virus was improving! Zinc was good at 73. Adrenals were better!

We were hoping that nutrition would have brought her estrogen, testosterone and DHEA up, but that did not happen. So, she was hypothyroid again. Therefore, we opted for a thyroid med called Nature-Throid. Our prayer was that she would only need this for 6 weeks and it would help her thyroid to kick in so the rest of her hormones will follow suite. She was also on a vitamin A supplement.

We were praying that this Nature-Throid would help her without doing damage to her stomach, since it is a medication. She had been dealing with some nausea because of it.

Psalm 84:11 was the scripture that was used to help Courtney. It says, "For the Lord God is a sun and shield; the Lord gives grace and glory; no good thing does He withhold from those who walk uprightly." (NAS) Another scripture says,

"Bless the Lord, O my soul, and forget none of His benefits; Who pardons all your iniquities; Who heals all your diseases;" Psalm 103:2-3 (NAS)

"Be anxious for nothing, but in everything by prayer and supplication with thanksgiving let your requests be made known to God. And the peace of God, which surpasses all comprehension, shall guard your hearts and your minds in Christ Jesus. Finally, brethren, whatever is true, whatever is honorable, whatever is right, whatever is pure, whatever is lovely, whatever is of good repute, if there is any excellence and if anything worthy of praise, let your mind dwell on these things" Philippians 4:6-8 (NAS)

February 23, Courtney had been diagnosed with streptococcal pharyngitis (strep throat). She was put on Pleo San Strep 10 drops twice daily for a week. It was suggested that she start using a new toothbrush in 3 days. She was to gargle with warm sea salt water. And take one teaspoon of colloidal silver twice daily.

March 29, 2018, her hemoglobin was high at 15.7 and hematocrit was high at 47.0. She continued to improve!

April 3, after watching a week-long docu-series from The Truth About Cancer, I started to wonder about heavy metals poisoning and vaccine injury. During this docu-series people gave their testimonies about how they cured their cancer in a year, for some people it took less time. I started to wonder when Courtney started seeing her NP. It had been a little over a year! Why had Courtney not completely healed? Could she be vaccine injured? Could heavy metals poisoning be her problem too?

April 16, 2018, Courtney's NP charted, "CBC is good. Thyroid is low. Reverse T3 is 14."

The supplements Courtney was taking were: Plexus ProBio5, Plexus XFactor multivitamin 2 capsules daily, Plexus Nerve 1 capsule twice daily, Plexus Ease 1 capsule daily, Monolaurin, Caprylic acid, Adrenal Support Plus capsules 1 capsule daily in the morning, Guna Liver 5 pellets before meals, Vitamin D3 2000 u/drop 2 drops under the tongue daily, Bio-Ae-Mulsion Forte (vitamin A) 10 drops under tongue daily for 3 days and then take 2 drops daily, PaxImmune 2 sprays under the tongue twice daily, and Progensa Mist 3 sprays topically daily, increase to 6 sprays on days 12 to 26.

It was recommended to stop bio-adaptogen and start iodine capsules 12.5 mg daily. She needed more probiotic therefore we increased the Probiotic 42.5 in the morning and in the evening to see if she tolerated it. It was suggested that we needed to consider an EBV series.

April 17, 2018, in January 2018 we retested her thyroid to see if the nutrition was working. Her body was not allowing us to add in vegetables as quickly as she needed. We made the decision to try a thyroid med for 6 weeks.

In February, Courtney got sick and we had to put off retesting. We tried treating her illness naturally but did not know about the mint depleting the effects of the homeopathic, according to her NP. We made the bad decision to put her on an antibiotic.

She finished the antibiotic, and I took her off the thyroid pill in March because her stomach was hurting so bad. At the doctor's office, Courtney told her NP that her stomach was hurting too bad to continue the thyroid pill and we took her off. To my surprise, her NP did not get mad. She simply said, "OK, we have other options." At this point Courtney decided to take her stand and she said, "No more chemicals!" I was so proud of her for standing up for herself! I was going to say the same thing, but she did not need me, she stood up for herself! Surprisingly, her NP said, "No problem, there's always something natural to try." I think what got her attention was not only that Courtney stood up for herself, but she also asked if she was still gaining weight. I said, "No, it has gradually been decreasing since the antibiotic."

Also, during muscle testing, her NP noticed a difference. At that point she said, "Even though she was taking two probiotics while on the antibiotic, the antibiotic almost DEPLETED ALL THE PROGRESS SHE HAD MADE."

Wow!!!

We had to combat the damage done from the antibiotic. She was taking 3 probiotics, 2 antifungals, and a liver detox along with a stronger iodine to increase her thyroid levels. Unfortunately, she was going through more detox.

The good news? Her immunity was up!

April 25, 2018, Courtney was put on a new probiotic called VSL#3. It had been causing her nausea. I looked at the ingredients and it had cornstarch in it! She is allergic to corn! Also, cornstarch feeds candida overgrowth! Why would anybody put cornstarch in a probiotic?!

I went to her doctor's office to get one of Courtney's probiotics and I asked the receptionist if he knew that the VSL#3 probiotic had cornstarch in it?

You should have seen the look on his face. He had no idea, and he knew it was bad! I think I may have left him a bit dazed and confused.

As I left, he said he was going to let the staff know. He said, "I don't know what we are going to do now. That probiotic has our highest CFUs!"

This, to me, was proof that folks are so focused on the highest CFUs that they cannot get past them to see the other ingredients! In my humble opinion, this is why ProBio5 works so well!

May 17, we were waiting for a call from the doctor's office. We were wondering about the possibility of Courtney having a vaccine injury from the Gardasil vaccine. I had taken a copy of her complete shot record to them so they could look it over. I always thought I was doing the right thing as her mother, like so many other parents.

I spoke with Courtney's NP about testing for heavy metals poisoning. I told her I could not afford more lab work at that time. She informed me that we could use muscle testing for heavy metals poisoning. We muscle tested her against her shot record and for possible heavy metals poisoning.

May 21, it had been confirmed that Courtney was a victim of vaccine injury by the Gardasil vaccine. We started her on a homeopathic that would reverse it. We were expecting a complete healing. Her NP was calling her a miracle!

June 21, she was halfway through the Gardasil homeopathic and she was becoming more alert and aware of her surroundings!

July 2, Courtney was finished with the Gardasil homeopathic! On July 11th she would go for muscle testing to see if she had any more of the Gardasil vaccine in her body. We were also going to test her for other vaccine injuries and for heavy metals poisoning. She was losing weight again and we were not sure why. Hopefully, the muscle testing would give us the answers. She had gone from 107.8 pounds to 104 pounds. She was terribly upset about this. I kept telling her that we need to focus on her gut health and her weight gain would follow.

July 9, as an LVN, who used to practice western medicine, I was once again amazed by alternative medicine!

Courtney's muscle testing confirmed that she was sensitive to mercury, gold and palladium as far as heavy metals goes. Therefore, she had one mercury filling that we needed to get removed and composite placed instead.

According to the muscle testing, EVERY SINGLE VACCINE SHE HAS EVER HAD WAS WORKING AGAINST HER! I was doing what I thought was best for her as her mother, and it was slowly killing her! We used to nick name Courtney our social butterfly when she was little. Since she was about 15 years old, she had been suffering from OCD (obsessive-compulsive disorder). During the muscle testing we asked her body, "Are the vaccines causing the OCD?" Her body told us yes!!!! She had been dealing with social anxiety for about a year. During the muscle testing we asked, "Are any of these vaccines affecting her brain?" Her body told us yes!!!!

According to muscle testing, her body was Gardasil free! Praise God!!!!

I asked her NP if she could help Courtney detox from the other vaccines and heavy metals poisoning and she said yes. As we were walking out of the room, her NP said, "I don't know the ingredients of vaccines." I was alarmed by this!

We started Courtney on their heavy metal detox protocol. Courtney had trouble with this protocol from the start.

August 3, 2018, it was recommended to decrease to 4 sprays once daily. Continue the alpha lipoic acid and heavy metals pill.

August 4, at home, Courtney had a major detox episode, or so I thought. She had an hour-long detox episode where she lost control of her body, was having vision and speech problems, and was feeling pressure in her chest. She was very tired after the episode, but she was feeling better. After the episode she said, "I would rather go through these tough times than to stay stuck." That's my girl! Courtney was past the episode and eating!

After her hour-long episode, I reported it to her NP. She wanted to see Courtney. Her NP confirmed that she had a seizure! As a nurse, I had never seen a seizure like what Courtney experienced.

According to her NP, Courtney was detoxing from all the vaccines too fast, therefore her dose was decreased. Courtney had also started her menstrual cycle the day before she had the seizure. During her past 2 cycles she had had a decrease in eating. This decrease is due to low progesterone, which was also a factor that prompted her seizure, according to her NP. She was already on a progesterone mist, but it was not enough. We put her on an oral progesterone instead.

August 6, 2018, it was charted that I called at 8:27 AM to see if Courtney's NP could call me back. I had done some research on the seizure Courtney had and was wondering about the vitamin D dose. I was wondering if the dose could be increased. I had also done some research about MTHFR and was wanting to discuss that with her NP as well.

At 9:36 AM the RN returned my call and instructed me to not increase the vitamin D because she was on the dose according to her lab results for the vitamin D. We would look at B12 and thyroid labs in 3 weeks and follow up in 4 weeks.

At 10:23 AM I called again to see if there was any way to increase Courtney's Progensa mist to 2-3 sprays daily until oral progesterone was started. I was not allowed to increase the mist.

We started Courtney on a prescription oral progesterone, and she started reacting to it. She started experiencing stomach pain, again. I looked at the ingredients and noticed peanut oil. Courtney is allergic to peanuts! I notified her NP and she said, "She has a very small peanut allergy." I said, "However, she is reacting. I'm taking her off and we will be patient with the progesterone mist."

August 18, since the seizure we had been on a rollercoaster ride with her health. Her anxiety, OCD, and social anxiety had been through the roof! She had been having chest tightness while eating, making eating EXCEEDINGLY difficult for her. She had been having a hard time swallowing her food, again. Her NP suggested pureeing her food. Her weight was down from 108.6 in May to 102.

I started her on Rescue Remedy and that was helping (thank you Jane Remington!). I had spoken with her NP and we took her off the pills that pull the toxins from her cells but left her on everything else. We added Diatomaceous Earth to help her detox instead of the pills.

All this had really messed with her brain. I felt like we just stirred up the heavy metals and vaccines and did not make any progress. I did start to suspicion MTHFR and brought it up to her NP and she said, "We are not even going to worry about that because we believe in epigenetics and not genetics." She said, "Besides that, she detoxed from the Gardasil vaccine just fine." Which was true! She also said since Plexus XFactor Plus is methylated then even if she did have it, it was not a problem! Her NP thought she simply had an EXTREMELY sensitive tummy and needed something not as strong. Hence, the Diatomaceous Earth. Plus, we realized the Gardasil vaccine was just one vaccine compared to ALL vaccines she had ever had in her life.

Since Courtney had a seizure, I decided to start researching about vaccines and the ingredients of them.

Chapter 12

Vaccines and Heavy Metals

Let's start with the DTP, one of the vaccines Courtney received. DTP is for Diphtheria, Tetanus and Pertussis. The DTP is a "whole cell" vaccine.

What is Diphtheria, Tetanus, and Pertussis? According to https://www.drugs.com/cg/dtp-vaccine.html

- Diphtheria is a serious disease that causes an infection and a thick covering in the nose and throat. This can cause breathing problems, paralysis (unable to move), heart failure, and even death.

- Tetanus (Lockjaw) happens when a wound like a cut gets infected with tetanus bacteria (germ) often found in dirt. The bacteria in the wound makes a poison that causes muscles all over the body to spasm (tighten) painfully. This can cause the jaw to "lock" so your child cannot open his/her mouth or swallow. Tetanus can also lead to death.

- Pertussis (Whooping Cough) causes bad coughing spells which make it hard for your child to eat, drink, or breathe. These coughing spells can last for weeks and can lead to pneumonia (lung infection), seizures (convulsions), brain damage, and death.

What are the ingredients of the DTP? According to https://www.rxlist.com/dtp-drug.htm#description

"Corynebacterium diphtheriae cultures are grown in a modified Mueller and Miller medium. Clostridium tetani cultures are grown in a peptone- based medium. Both toxins are detoxified with FORMALDEHYDE. The detoxified materials are separately purified by serial ammonium sulfate fractionation and diafiltration.

The pertussis vaccine component is derived from Bordetella pertussis cultures grown on blood-free Bordet Gengou media. The pertussis organisms are harvested and inactivated with THIMEROSAL and resuspended in physiological saline and THIMEROSAL.

The toxoids are adsorbed to ALUMINUM potassium sulfate (alum). The adsorbed diphtheria and tetanus toxoids are combined with pertussis vaccine concentrate and diluted to a final volume using sterile phosphate-buffered physiological saline. Each 0.5 mL dose contains, by assay, not more than 0.17 mg of ALUMINUM and not more than 100 µg (0.02%)

of residual FORMALDEHYDE. THIMEROSAL (MERCURY derivative) 1:10,000 is added as a preservative.

Each 0.5 mL dose is formulated to contain 6.7 Lf of diphtheria toxoid and 5 Lf of tetanus toxoid (both toxoids induce at least 2 units of antitoxin per mL in the guinea pig potency test).

The total human immunizing dose (the first three 0.5 mL doses administered) contains an estimate of 12 units of pertussis vaccine (4 protective units per single dose). [2] The potency of the pertussis component of each lot of DTP (diphtheria and tetanus toxoids and pertussis vaccine absorbed usp) is tested in a mouse protection test.

At the time when Connaught Laboratories, Inc. (CLI) DTP (diphtheria and tetanus toxoids and pertussis vaccine adsorbed usp) vaccine is used to reconstitute ActHIB ® or OmniHIB, each single dose of the 0.5 mL mixture is formulated to contain 6.7 Lf of diphtheria toxoid, 5 Lf of tetanus toxoid, an estimate of 4 protective units of pertussis vaccine, 10 µg of purified capsular polysaccharide conjugated to 24 µg of inactivated tetanus toxoid, and 8.5% of SUCROSE." (emphasis added)

According to https://www.scarymommy.com/truth-vaccine-injuries/

"Dr. Moore tells Scary Mommy that in her entire time practicing — a whopping 14 years — she has seen two vaccine-injured patients, and one during her residency. That teen was injured by an earlier formulation, now changed, of a DTP (now DTaP) vaccine, which caused encephalitis as an infant. Another child, she says, developed "idiopathic thrombocytopenia purpura (ITP) about ten days or so following his MMR vaccine. Even though [he] recovered completely within a week of the ITP, that qualifies as a vaccine injury as per the CDC Vaccine Injury Table."

What is Tdap?

Tdap is still Tetanus, Diphtheria, and Pertussis. Tdap is a booster given at age 11 that offers continued protection from those diseases for adolescents and adults. It contains inactivated (not live) form of the toxin produced by the bacteria that cause the three diseases. Vaccines that are not live are inactivated (contain microbes killed by chemicals, heat, or radiation), subunits (contain only part of the microbe), toxoids (inactivated toxins), or conjugate (a subunit linked to a toxoid). The "a" in Tdap stands for acellular. But since immunity to pertussis also wears off during childhood, a weaker form of the pertussis vaccine has been added to the booster to make the vaccine Tdap. Tdap is different than the DTaP vaccine (Diphtheria, Tetanus, and Whooping cough), which is given to infants and children in five doses, starting at 2 months of age. Tdap is only for those above the age of 7 years.

What are the ingredients of the Tdap?

According to https://vaccineingredients.net/vaccines/tdap-adacel

"In addition to the live, attenuated or inactive virus, pathogen or toxoid, the Tdap (Adacel) vaccine contains the following ingredients:

- ALUMINUM phosphate
- FORMALDEHYDE
- 2-phenoxyethanol (a central nervous system depressant)
- Stainer-Scholte medium
- Casamino acids
- Dimethyl-beta-cyclodextrin
- Glutaraldehyde (disinfectant)
- modified Mueller-Miller casamino acid medium without beef heart infusion
- AMMONIUM sulfate
- modified Mueller's growth medium
    (emphasis added)

What is polio?

According to https://www.mayoclinic.org/diseases-conditions/polio/symptoms-causes/syc-20376512

"Polio is a contagious viral illness that in its most severe form causes nerve injury leading to paralysis, difficulty breathing and sometimes death."

What are the ingredients of the polio vaccine?

According to https://vaccineingredients.net/vaccines/polio-ipv-ipol

"The Polio (IPV – Ipol) vaccine contains the following ingredients:

- Eagle MEM modified medium
- Calf bovine serum (calf blood)
- M-199 without calf bovine serum
- Vero cells (a continuous line of MONKEY KIDNEY CELLS)
- phenoxyethanol (ANTIFREEZE)- toxic to ALL cells and capable of blocking immune response
- FORMALDEHYDE (used to embalm corpses; poisonous if ingested; probable carcinogen; suspected gastrointestinal (GI), liver, immune system, nerve, reproductive system, and respiratory poison; linked to leukemia, brain, colon and lymphatic cancer)
- Neomycin (antibiotic)
- Streptomycin (antibiotic)
- Polymyxin B
(emphasis added)

According to https://thetruthaboutvaccines.com/polio-vaccine-cancer/

"In order to grow large quantities of the poliovirus, scientists needed to use Rhesus monkey kidney cells, which carried many different viruses. As a result, their polio vaccine became contaminated with a cancer-causing virus carried by these monkeys. This vaccine was given to almost 100 million people.

The virus found in this particular polio vaccine was SV40, or simian virus. It is present in human tumors, and research has established it to be a contributing factor in the rise of many types of cancer, including mesothelioma, bone, and brain cancer.

When the government became aware of this, it was downplayed for fear the public would stop accepting vaccination."

According to https://holisticlifemama.com/2016/01/31/the-truth-about-polio/

"It seems that the public has been misled for decades about how dangerous polio is.   In over

90% of cases, polio is symptomless. Less than 5% of those with polio became seriously ill. Most symptoms included a slight fever, headache, sore throat, and vomiting. (The recovery time was 24 – 72 hrs.). Once recovered, the person then had lifetime immunity to Polio. Paralysis from the condition was known to be extremely rare – Less than 2%, with half of those completely recovering from the paralysis. In most people with a healthy immune system, polio does not generate any symptoms.

During the times of the epidemic of polio in the US scientists were discussing the fact that many commonly used neurotoxins such as lead, arsenic and DDT caused lesions of neurological tissues to manifest, which were identical to that of polio. Around this time many alternative doctors were able to reverse polio symptoms in patients by detoxification procedures.

In 1955, the AMA instructed doctors to no longer call polio by its name but to diagnose all polio-like paralysis as MS, Guillain-Barre or Acute Flaccid Paralysis."

According to https://www.westonaprice.org/health-topics/vaccinations/polio-vaccines-medical-triumph-or-medical-mishap/

"In 1996, Michele Carbone, a molecular pathologist at Loyola University Medical Center, was able to detect SV40 in 38 percent of patients with bone cancer and in 58 percent of those with mesothelioma, a deadly type of lung cancer.[1] By April 2001, sixty-two papers from thirty laboratories around the world had reported SV40 in human tissues and tumors, including pituitary and thyroid cancers.[1] Dr. Hilleman later admitted—on tape—that Merck knew that the vaccines were contaminated but continued to dispense them to the public anyway.[26]

The polio vaccines used today supposedly do not contain SV40, yet one must consider the fact that it took the CDC fifty years to be forthright and admit that their recommended polio vaccines had been tainted.[27] Until recently, the agency's admission that as many as thirty million Americans could be at risk for developing cancer due to SV40-contaminated polio vaccines could be found on the CDC website; the CDC later removed this information, but it can still be found in archived format.[28]"

The Sabine polio vaccine contains a live virus. Live viruses wreak havoc on your brain cells.

What is Hib?

According to https://www.drugs.com/cg/hib-vaccine.html

"Hib is Haemophilus influenzae type b (Hib) infection. Hib is a common bacterial infection that spreads when a person coughs, sneezes, or shares utensils."

According to https://kidshealth.org/en/parents/hib-vaccine.html

"Haemophilus influenzae type b bacteria (Hib) were the leading cause of meningitis in children younger than 5 years old until the Hib vaccine became available. It also used to be a common cause of infections in the ears, lungs, blood, skin, and joints in children."

What are the ingredients of the Hib vaccine?

According to https://vaccineingredients.net/vaccines/hib-acthib

"In addition to the live, attenuated or inactive virus, pathogen or toxoid, the Hib (ActHIB) vaccine contains the following ingredients:

- Sodium chloride
- Modified Mueller and Miller medium (the culture medium contains milk-derived raw materials [casein derivatives])
- FORMALDEHYDE (used to embalm corpses; poisonous if ingested; probable carcinogen; suspected gastrointestinal (GI), liver, immune system, nerve, reproductive system, and respiratory poison; linked to leukemia, brain, colon and lymphatic cancer)
- SUCROSE (sugar)"
(emphasis added)

MMR stands for Measles, Mumps and Rubella.

What is Measles, Mumps and Rubella?

According to https://www.stanfordchildrens.org/en/topic/default?id=measles-mumps-and-rubella-mmr-90-P02250

- Measles. Measles is an infection caused by a virus. It starts with cold-like symptoms including runny nose; inflamed, red eyes; cough; and fever. A rash that starts on the face and then develops on the body follows 2 to 4 days later.

- Mumps. Mumps is also caused by a virus. It mainly affects the glands. Symptoms are swollen saliva-producing glands in the neck, fever, headache, and muscle aches.

- Rubella (German measles). Rubella is an infection from a virus. It causes mild fever and rash in infants and children. Pregnant women who get rubella have an increased chance of having babies with birth defects.

What are the ingredients of the MMR?

According to https://vaccineingredients.net/vaccines/mmr-mmr-ii

"In addition to the live, attenuated or inactive virus, pathogen or toxoid, the MMR (MMR-II) vaccine contains the following ingredients:

- CHICK EMBRYO CELL culture
- WI-38 HUMAN diploid LUNG fibroblasts (diploid means cells originated from ABORTED fetal tissues)
- vitamins

- amino acids
- fetal bovine serum (baby cow blood)
- SUCROSE (sugar)
- Glutamate (MSG), excitotoxin-a neurotoxin, being studied for mutagenic, teratogenic, and reproductive effect, and a suspected carcinogen
- Recombinant human albumin (recombinant DNA molecules are DNA molecules formed by laboratory methods) (albumin is blood)
- Neomycin (antibiotic)
- Sorbitol (sugar)
- Hydrolyzed gelatin
- Sodium phosphate
- Sodium chloride"
(emphasis added)

Measles, mumps and rubella are all viral infections that caused widespread illness in the past. Vaccines to prevent each disease were first developed in the 1960s and then combined to form the MMR vaccine in the 1970s. The MMR contains live viruses. Live viruses wreak havoc on your brain cells. When two or four live viruses are given together, the risk of catching any opportunistic germ a person is exposed to or developing a chronic lifetime infection increases dramatically. The MMR vaccine contains two live viruses that are known to suppress the immune system for months.

Vaccines have not been safety tested in combination with each other, only individually. Nor have the effects of the entire cumulative load of vaccines EVER been safety tested! In some people the virus is not killed off, but instead takes up permanent residence in a person's internal organs. Autopsies routinely find live measles viruses embedded in organs and even the brain.

You can go to https://www.merck.com/product/usa/pi_circulars/m/mmr_ii/mmr_ii_pi.pdf and see that Merck's MMRII insert states right on the first page: ("Rubella Virus Vaccine Live), the Wistar RA 27/3 strain of live attenuated rubella virus propagated in WI-38 human diploid lung fibroblasts."

Translation?

First be aware that the development of the rubella vaccine in the United States involved not one, but 28 abortions (27 abortions to isolate the virus and one more abortion to culture the vaccine.) The vaccine's strain is called RA 27/3, meaning R=rubella, 27=27th fetus tested, 3=3rd tissue explanted. We know the single aborted human was a girl.

To produce a "live" vaccine such as MMR (measles/mumps/rubella), the virus is passed through animal tissue several times to reduce its potency. Measles virus is passed through chick embryos and the rubella virus through the dissected organs of aborted human fetuses.

We know that live virus vaccines such as measles, mumps, rubella (MMR) can survive and remain dormant for years in the host's body, waiting for opportunities to erupt into more serious diseases like rheumatoid arthritis (RA), multiple sclerosis (MS), lupus, and cancer when the host is stressed, this is known as provocation disease. Courtney, our current generation and our future generations will pay a huge price for this misguided immunosuppression.

Courtney and I highly recommend the book, *Recaging the Beast* by Jane Remington to explain more. It can be purchased on Amazon.com.

What is (OPV) Oral Polio Vaccine?

According to https://vaxxter.com/oral-polio-vaccines-causing-polio/

"OPV is still used worldwide today. The OPV contains three live but attenuated (weakened) viruses. They pass through the body and are eliminated in the feces. The viruses can regain virulence in the environment and return to their original virulent forms, leading to paralysis.

Oral poliovirus vaccines (OPV) are used in third world countries in an attempt to eradicate polio the last vestiges of polioviruses on the planet. There are different types of oral poliovirus vaccine, which may contain one, two, or all three different attenuated serotypes.

The process of attenuation is the serial passage of a virus through tissues to weaken it. The scientific literature admits that attenuation is a haphazard process that relies on trial and error. It is known that the attenuated viruses may revert back to full virulence under specified conditions.

So, the problem with continuing to use the oral vaccine is that the viruses in the vaccine are reverting to active virulence and will continually cause new disease."

According to https://childrenshealthdefense.org/news/childrens-health/polio-vaccination-still-causing-polio-after-all-these-years/

"Vaccine researchers have long known that these OPV-derived viruses can themselves cause polio, particularly when they get "loose in the environment." In settings with poor sanitation and iffy hygiene, the vaccine viruses can easily "find their way into water sources, and onto contaminated hands or foods," where they can then launch a self-perpetuating chain of transmission. Researchers concede that an OPV virus "can very rapidly regain its strength if it starts spreading on its own," acquiring "mutations that make it basically indistinguishable from the wild-type virus." In other words, there is no meaningful difference between a wild and OPV-derived poliovirus "in terms of virulence and in terms of how the virus spreads."

According to https://www.westonaprice.org/health-topics/vaccinations/polio-vaccines-medical-triumph-or-medical-mishap/

"In 1963, the U.S. replaced Salk's IPV vaccine with an attenuated (weakened, not killed) oral polio vaccine (OPV) developed by American physician and microbiologist, Albert Sabin. As a live virus vaccine, it, too, was (and continues to be) capable of giving its recipients polio. Not only can OPV trigger vaccine-strain polio in recipients, it can also cause polio in those who come in contact with recently vaccinated individuals due to shedding of live vaccine-strain poliovirus in bodily fluids.[12] In validation of this very theory, Dr. Salk testified before a Senate subcommittee in 1977 that the oral polio vaccine had caused most of the polio cases in the U.S. since the early 1960s.[17]

Today, the U.S. has reverted to using an updated version of Salk's "killed" IPV vaccine. Meanwhile, Sabin's live OPV vaccine continues to be widely used in other parts of the world, and particularly in lower-income countries, as it is less expensive to produce."

What is the flu?

According to https://www.mayoclinic.org/diseases-conditions/flu/symptoms-causes/syc-20351719

"Influenza is a viral infection that attacks your respiratory system — your nose, throat and lungs. Influenza is commonly called the flu."

What are the ingredients of the flu vaccine?

According to this vaccine insert https://www.fda.gov/media/135432/download

"Inactivated influenza vaccine prepared from virus propagated in the allantoic cavity of embryonated hens' eggs inoculated with a specific type of influenza virus. A SQUALENE based oil-in-water emulsion.

Each of the strains is harvested and clarified separately by centrifugation and filtration prior to inactivation with FORMALDEHYDE. The surface antigens, hemagglutinin, and neuraminidase, are obtained from the influenza virus particle by further centrifugation in the presence of cetyltrimethylammonium bromide (CTAB). Each 0.5 mL dose contains 15 mcg of hemagglutinin (HA) from each of the four recommended influenza strains and MF59C.1 adjuvant (9.75 mg SQUALENE, 1.175 mg of POLYSORBATE 80, 1.175 mg of sorbitan trioleate, 0.66 mg of sodium citrate dihydrate and 0.04 mg of citric acid monohydrate) at pH 6.9-7.7. FLUAD QUADRIVALENT may contain trace amounts of NEOMYCIN ($\leq$ 0.02 mcg by calculation), kanamycin ($\leq$ 0.03 mcg by calculation) and HYDROCORTISONE ($\leq$ 0.005 ng by calculation) which are used during the initial stages of manufacture, as well as residual egg protein (ovalbumin) ($\leq$ 1.0 mcg), FORMALDEHYDE ($\leq$ 10 mcg) or CTAB ($\leq$ 18 mcg). FLUAD QUADRIVALENT does not contain a preservative. The syringe, syringe plunger stopper and tip caps are not made with natural rubber latex." (emphasis added)

- Squalene-an adjuvant so toxic that a single dose injected into rats causes them to develop rheumatoid arthritis (RA)
- Polysorbate 80-an emulsifier and known carcinogen in animals

- Hydrocortisone-steroid

Thimerosal is still used in multi-dose vials of influenza vaccines. Thimerosal is a preservative that is almost fifty percent mercury. In 1998 it was banned in over the counter (OTC) drugs because "safety and efficacy have not been established for the ingredients." It inhibits phagocytes, one of the most vital immune defenses in the blood. Still present in DPT, DTaP, Hib, Varicella, and Inactivated Polio Vaccine (IPV). Flu vaccines containing thimerosal contain 250 times above the level identified as hazardous waste! Known to induce breaks in DNA.

What is Hepatitis B?

Hepatitis B is primarily transmitted sexually or through sharing of needles among injection drug users. The hepatitis B virus (HBV) can also be transmitted to infants at birth, if the mother is a carrier. But screening to identify infected pregnant women is done routinely, and an alternative effective treatment has long been available for infants born to carriers. So, is the Hep B vaccine necessary for all infants?

According to https://childrenshealthdefense.org/news/cdcs-recommendation-for-hepatitis-b-vaccination-in-infants-are-there-more-risks-than-benefits/

"Transmission of the virus occurs through infected blood or other bodily fluids. Subpopulations at highest risk therefore include sexually active individuals, injection drug users, health care workers, and children who are born to infected mothers or otherwise come into prolonged close contact with infected household members. Mother-to-infant transmission usually occurs during birth. The vast majority of children in the US today are not at significant risk of hepatitis B infection.) Persons considered at "substantial risk" included various categories of health care workers, gay men, illicit injectable drug users, recipients of certain blood products, household and sexual contacts of HBV carriers, Alaskan Eskimos, immigrants or refugees from countries where HBV is highly endemic, and prison inmates. The stated reason why the CDC wanted to vaccinate all infants was not because all infants were at risk of infection, but simply because its strategy to vaccinate high-risk populations was failing. However, the strategy has not lowered the incidence of hepatitis B, primarily because vaccinating persons engaged in high-risk behaviors, lifestyles, or occupations before they become infected generally has not been feasible." Infants, of course, do not engage in those high-risk behaviors. The CDC's reasoning was simply that, since adults tended for various reasons to not get the vaccine, it would eliminate the choice by vaccinating everyone at birth, regardless of individual risk."

What are the ingredients of the Hepatitis B vaccine?

According to https://childrenshealthdefense.org/news/cdcs-recommendation-for-hepatitis-b-vaccination-in-infants-are-there-more-risks-than-benefits/

"Aluminum—a known neurotoxin—as an "adjuvant". Mercury, another known neurotoxin. Merck's Recombivax HB, instead contained viral proteins that were genetically engineered, manufactured by cloning the virus's genetic coding for HBsAg into "recombinant" yeast. Thimerosal is still used in hepatitis B vaccines licensed for use in infants still contain aluminum.

What are the ingredients of the Hepatitis B vaccine?

According to https://vaccineingredients.net/vaccines/hep-b-engerix-b

"In addition to the live, attenuated or inactive virus, pathogen or toxoid, the Hep B (Engerix-B) vaccine contains the following ingredients:

- ALUMINUM hydroxide
- YEAST protein
- Sodium chloride

- Disodium phosphate dihydrate (additive and emulsifier)
- Sodium dihydrogen phosphate dihydrate"
  (emphasis added)

Courtney received Menactra, which is the meningococcal vaccine. The Meningococcal vaccine is for meningitis.

What is meningitis?

Meningitis is an inflammation of the fluid and membranes (meninges) surrounding your brain and spinal cord.

According to
https://www.drugs.com/menactra.html

"Meningococcal disease can spread from one person to another through small droplets of saliva that are expelled into the air when an infected person coughs or sneezes. The bacteria can also be passed through contact with objects the infected person has touched, such as a door handle or other surface. The bacteria can also be passed through kissing or sharing a drinking glass or eating utensil with an infected person."

What are the ingredients of Menactra, the meningitis vaccine?

According to the Menactra package insert
https://www.fda.gov/media/75619/download

"Menactra is a sterile, intramuscularly administered vaccine that contains N meningitidis serogroup A, C, Y and W-135 capsular polysaccharide antigens individually conjugated to diphtheria toxoid protein. N meningitidis A, C, Y and W-135 strains are cultured on Mueller Hinton agar (3) and grown in Watson Scherp (4) media containing casamino acid. The polysaccharides are extracted from the N meningitidis cells and purified by centrifugation, DETERGENT precipitation, alcohol precipitation, solvent extraction and diafiltration. To prepare the polysaccharides for conjugation, they are depolymerized, derivatized, and purified by diafiltration. Diphtheria toxin is derived from Corynebacterium diphtheriae grown in modified culture medium containing hydrolyzed casein (5) and is detoxified using FORMALDEHYDE. The diphtheria toxoid protein is purified by AMMONIUM sulfate fractionation and diafiltration. The derivatized polysaccharides are covalently linked to diphtheria toxoid and purified by serial diafiltration. The four meningococcal components, present as individual serogroup-specific glycoconjugates, compose the final formulated vaccine. No preservative or adjuvant is added during manufacture. Each 0.5 mL dose may contain residual amounts of FORMALDEHYDE of less than 2.66 mcg (0.000532%), by calculation. Potency of Menactra is determined by quantifying the amount of each polysaccharide antigen that is conjugated to diphtheria toxoid protein and the amount of unconjugated polysaccharide present. Menactra is manufactured as a sterile, clear to slightly turbid liquid. Each 0.5 mL dose of vaccine is formulated in sodium phosphate buffered isotonic sodium chloride solution to contain 4 mcg each of meningococcal A, C, Y and W-135 polysaccharides conjugated to approximately 48 mcg of diphtheria toxoid protein carrier. The vial stopper is not made with natural rubber latex." (emphasis added)

What is Human Papilloma Virus (HPV)?

According to https://www.healthline.com/health/human-papillomavirus-infection

"Human papillomavirus (HPV) is a viral infection that's passed between people through skin-to-skin contact. There are over 100 varieties of HPV, more than 40 of which are passed through sexual contact and can affect your genitals, mouth, or throat.

According to the Centers for Disease Control and Prevention, HPV is the most common sexually transmitted infection (STI).

It is so common that most sexually active people will get some variety of it at some point, even if they have few sexual partners.

Some cases of genital HPV infection may not cause any health problems. However, some types of HPV can lead to the development of genital warts and even cancers of the cervix, anus, and throat."

When I was in nursing school, it was taught to us that the Gardasil vaccine was used to PREVENT cervical cancer. I did not want Courtney to have cervical cancer. So, the next time I took her to her pediatrician, I requested it. That's right, I requested it. The nurse said, "Ok." She did not ask me if I was sure. She did not try giving me any education at all. I wish I would have done my own research. However, I should have been able to trust her pediatrician's office and my nursing college instructor, right?

I specifically asked for the Gardasil vaccine because that is what we were educated on in nursing school.

According to https://www.drugs.com/gardasil.html

"Important Information

You should not receive a Gardasil 9 booster vaccine if you have had a life-threatening allergic reaction after the first shot.

Gardasil 9 vaccine will not protect against sexually transmitted diseases such as chlamydia, gonorrhea, herpes, HIV, syphilis, and trichomoniasis.

You may feel faint during the first 15 minutes after receiving this vaccine. Some people have had seizure-like reactions after receiving this vaccine."

According to https://www.healthline.com/health/sexually-transmitted-diseases/hpv-vaccine-pros-and-cons#pros

"The HPV vaccine can protect against HPV types 16 and 18, both of which can lead to certain cancers."

What are the ingredients in the Gardasil vaccine?

According to
https://www.fda.gov/media/74350/download

"GARDASIL, Human Papillomavirus Quadrivalent (Types 6, 11, 16, and 18) Vaccine, Recombinant, is a non-infectious recombinant quadrivalent vaccine prepared from the purified virus-like particles (VLPs) of the major capsid (L1) protein of HPV Types 6, 11, 16, and 18. The L1 proteins are produced by separate fermentations in recombinant SACCHAROMYCES CEREVISIAE and self-assembled into VLPs. The fermentation process involves growth of S. CEREVISIAE on chemically defined fermentation media which include vitamins, amino acids, mineral salts, and carbohydrates. The VLPs are released from the YEAST cells by cell disruption and purified by a series of chemical and physical

215

methods. The purified VLPs are adsorbed on preformed ALUMINUM-containing adjuvant (Amorphous ALUMINUM Hydroxyphosphate Sulfate). The quadrivalent HPV VLP vaccine is a sterile liquid suspension that is prepared by combining the adsorbed VLPs of each HPV type and additional amounts of the ALUMINUM-containing adjuvant and the final purification buffer. GARDASIL is a sterile suspension for intramuscular administration. Each 0.5-mL dose contains approximately 20 mcg of HPV 6 L1 protein, 40 mcg of HPV 11 L1 protein, 40 mcg of HPV 16 L1 protein, and 20 mcg of HPV 18 L1 protein. Each 0.5-mL dose of the vaccine contains approximately 225 mcg of ALUMINUM (as Amorphous ALUMINUM Hydroxyphosphate Sulfate adjuvant), 9.56 mg of sodium chloride, 0.78 mg of L-histidine, 50 mcg of POLYSORBATE 80, 35 mcg of sodium borate, < 7 mcg YEAST protein/dose, and water for injection. The product does not contain a preservative or antibiotics." (emphasis added)

Saccharomyces cerevisiae is the yeast they use to brew beer. Therefore, injecting Gardasil is just like injecting beer into the brain. It is going to cause inflammation in the brain which will in turn decrease blood flow to the brain. This was why Courtney was so pale and why the hormone test stated that she was premenopausal. Most of our hormonal system is in the brain.

Since we are on the subject of vaccines, do you remember the written instructions Courtney's first pediatrician gave to me when she was a newborn? Remember he told me to give her Tylenol before and after taking her for vaccines. Since then, I learned from Dr. Tenpenny's website, Vaxxter.com, that Tylenol and vaccines do not mix! Glutathione is naturally produced in our bodies and much of it is in our brains. When glutathione is in short supply, we suffer. In other words, not having enough glutathione places our bodies at serious risk of an adverse reaction by vaccines. You can read more about this here https://vaxxter.com/is-acetaminophen-fanning-the-flames-of-vaccine-injury/

Continuing with ingredients, and what we have learned about toxic heavy metals, remember the Mylanta that Courtney was on in the hospital? Did you know that aluminum hydroxide is in Mylanta? It is a toxic heavy metal in the body!

According to https://www.healmindbody.com/aluminum-sources-environment-detox/

One dose of Mylanta contains 200 milligrams of toxic aluminum.

She was also on Tums.

According to https://dailyhealthpost.com/liver-aluminum-detox/

Aluminum is toxic in the body and too much of it can cause symptoms like headaches, nausea, fever, fatigue, and abdominal pain.

We had been trying to stop the nausea and abdominal pain! Instead, we were making it worse!

Since the liver is one of the body's filtration systems, everything you take in goes through it and some, unfortunately, stays within your tissues.

Therefore, Courtney had to detox from these medications as well. And doctor's hand it out like it is not a problem!

Please be aware that many vaccines also have peanut oil as an ingredient. Peanut Oil is a hidden and non-stated ingredient in children's vaccines. Have you ever wondered where all the peanut allergies are coming from these days? Aflatoxin, a dangerous mycotoxin produced by Aspergillus flavus mold, is often found on peanuts and can cause anaphylaxis. Anaphylaxis is a serious allergic reaction that is rapid in onset and may cause death.

I was getting concerned about parasites as well. Why else would she keep hitting walls over this 3 ½ year period and having such a hard time gaining weight? She told me, "Mom, I'm ready to go back to being myself again!" She would make such good progress and we would think we had found the right combination of food and supplements for her and then she would hit a wall.

Do you remember in this book when I requested that you pay attention to Courtney's vital signs? The reason for that was because I had discovered that heavy metal poisoning was what was causing Courtney's vital signs to fluctuate like they were. Our bodies do not know how to react to heavy metal poisoning. Toxic heavy metals are a foreign invader to humans.

Remember in this book when I mentioned that George Bush was the president when Courtney was born? In 1986 he signed the National Childhood Vaccine Injury Act. This act took away ALL liability of vaccine injuries from physician's and vaccine manufacturers. If your child suffers, it is ONLY your fault and at your expense. This act needs to be repealed.

Chapter 13

The Amalgam Removal

I felt like she needed a brain detox from the vaccines and heavy metals that were in her brain. I was looking at either TRS (she had muscle tested favorably to this, but her NP was extremely cautious) or Dr. Daniel Pompa's brain phase detox (I had not talked to her NP about this yet).

August 30, 2018, Courtney and I both were struggling with spiritual warfare.

Remember when she was in the hospital and her lab work indicated microcytic anemia? Microcytic anemia is also an indication of lead toxicity!

October 5, 2018, I made an appointment to go to Evergreen, Colorado to get Courtney's amalgam filling removed and refilled with composite.

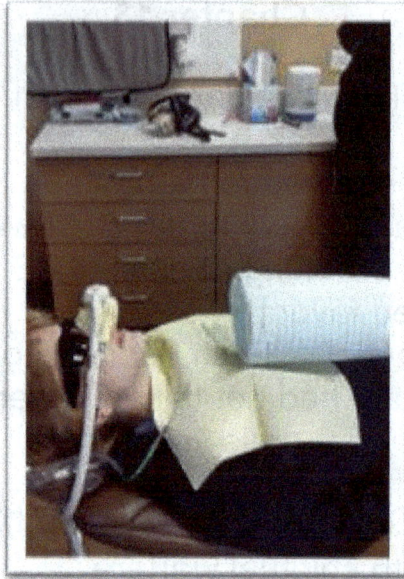

Did you know that each amalgam filling is 50% mercury? And, every time you chew your food, brush your teeth and drink something warm, you are causing that mercury to vapor up to your brain! Watching this video is an excellent visual of what happens. https://www.youtube.com/watch?v=9L9SF2ALrl l

Mercury is one of the most poisonous substances known. Minute amounts can cause nerve damage. It is toxic to the central nervous system (CNS) and not easily eliminated from the body. It has an affinity for the brain, gut, liver, bone marrow, and kidneys. Symptoms of mercury poisoning are like those of autism.

Mercury also kills beneficial bacteria in the gut stimulating the growth of yeast, and rapidly crosses the placental barrier and accumulates in a fetus at even higher levels than the mother!

There is NO safe dose for mercury in a human.

October 15, 2018, immediately after Courtney's amalgam filling was removed and she stood up to leave, she needed to hang on to me and I thought it was the anesthetic. Once we got to Idaho Springs and she started waking up from the anesthetic, she was still having a hard time walking and she was complaining of being dizzy. She needed assistance and was still walking awfully slow. I thought a good night's sleep was what she needed.

The next morning, she was still not walking any better and still complaining of dizziness. I started getting concerned. The hostess at the cabin said it was probably altitude sickness. I had never heard of altitude sickness, so I asked her what the symptoms were. She spouted off the symptoms and everything correlated except for her manner of walking.

After we were home, her lower back and legs were getting even more stiff. I added high doses of vitamin C, Plexus Nerve, and colloidal silver to her usual supplement regimen. The next morning, she woke up too stiff to even walk. I started rolling her to and from the bathroom in a rolling desk chair.

I contacted her temporary coach with Dr. Daniel Pompa via email. She and I had emailed back and forth before the trip and we had figured out a regimen that I could do on my own for Courtney that would involve Plexus supplements, Young Living essential oils, nutrition, and Kangen water. She would be starting some of Dr. Pompa's supplements as well. I was not able to afford coaching therefore, she helped me temporarily via email to get Courtney started on Dr. Pompa's supplements, his Binder and Cytodetox. We prayed that these two supplements would get her to walking again. Then he had a brain phase Courtney would do as well.

Courtney had become so stiff that we had to borrow a wheelchair.

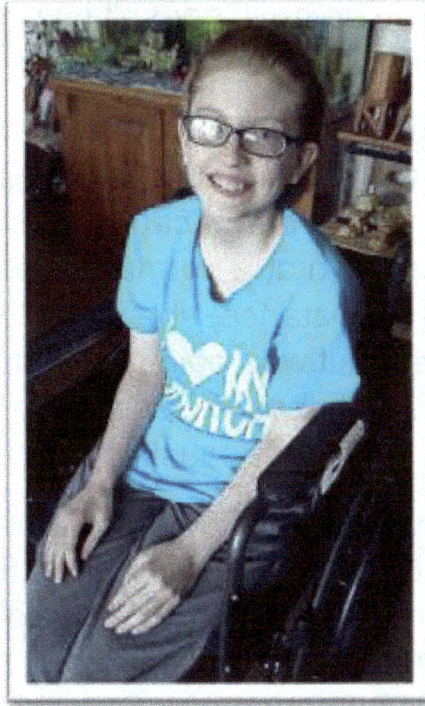

November 7, 2018, she was getting her balance back! She was getting color back in her face, her eyes were getting clear, and the dark circles around her eyes were almost gone! She had also been energetic and giggly, instead of tired and frustrated. Her OCD seemed to be lifting too!

November 11, 2018, Courtney walked across the room by herself! I stayed with her as stand by assistance. Her balance needed to improve. She went slow because she was having a hard time putting one foot in front of the other. Almost as if her feet were heavy.

She said, "The devil doesn't like you being my mom."

November 28, 2018, Courtney saw Dr. Jack Mustard for the first time. He is a holistic chiropractor. I took her because she was unable to walk on her own at a normal pace. When walking, with assistance, she would walk awfully slow and it was painful to her. After her first visit, she still needed assistance, but walking was no longer causing pain!

December 1, 2018, Courtney's 3rd appointment with Dr. Jack Mustard. She started out doing 5 minutes on a machine called Gadget Fit and she complained that her lower back was still bothering her. She did 20 minutes with no problem! She had gone from a wheelchair fulltime to a walker fulltime!

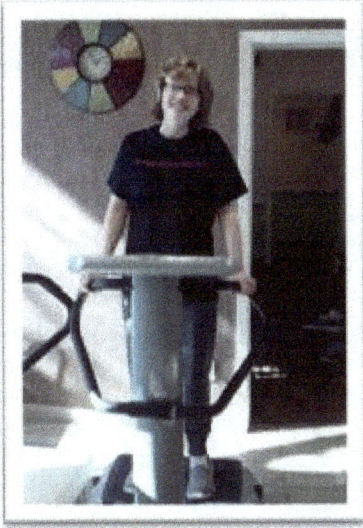

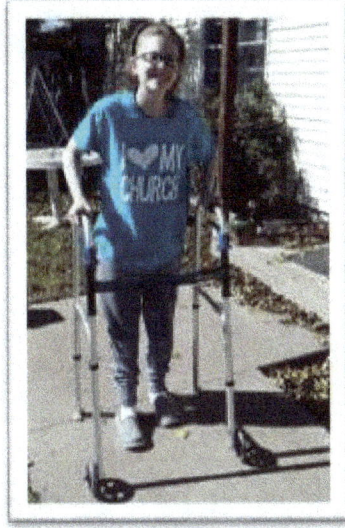

December 4, 2018, Courtney started walking! She walked down the hallway of the house all by herself! She was stiff and had to concentrate extremely hard, but she did it!

December 5, 2018, she did a home twenty-four-hour urine toxic metals test using DMSA as the provoking agent. It showed that she was heavy metal poisoned from ten different heavy metals. Aluminum, arsenic, barium, cesium, lead, mercury, nickel, thallium, tungsten, and uranium.

TOXIC METALS PER CREATININE			TOXIC METALS PER 24 HOURS			
	RESULT µg/g creat	REFERENCE INTERVAL	RESULT µg/24 hour	REFERENCE INTERVAL	WITHIN REFERENCE	OUTSIDE REFERENCE
Aluminum (Al)	3.4	35	2.7	39		
Antimony (Sb)	< dl	0.2	< dl	0.2		
Arsenic (As)	12	80	9.3	92		
Barium (Ba)	7.6	7	6.1	7		
Beryllium (Be)	< dl	1	< dl	1		
Bismuth (Bi)	< dl	4	< dl	4		
Cadmium (Cd)	< dl	1	< dl	1.3		
Cesium (Cs)	3.3	10	2.6	10		
Gadolinium (Gd)	< dl	0.4	< dl	2.0		
Lead (Pb)	5.8	2	4.7	2		
Mercury (Hg)	1	4	0.8	4		
Nickel (Ni)	1.2	10	0.9	10		
Palladium (Pd)	< dl	0.1	< dl	0.3		
Platinum (Pt)	< dl	0.1	< dl	0.2		
Tellurium (Te)	< dl	0.5	< dl	0.5		
Thallium (Tl)	0.3	0.3	0.2	0.4		
Thorium (Th)	< dl	0.03	< dl	0.03		
Tin (Sn)	< dl	5	< dl	4		
Tungsten (W)	0.1	0.4	0.09	0.4		
Uranium (U)	0.5	0.04	0.4	1		

URINE CREATININE							
	RESULT mg/24 hr	REFERENCE INTERVAL	-2SD	-1SD	MEAN	+1SD	+2SD

When we received Courtney's results, I was shocked! I never expected this many! I knew I had more researching to do to figure out where these heavy metals were coming from. When I shared the results of this test with other knowledgeable people, I was informed about climate engineering. To learn more about climate engineering I recommend this website https://www.geoengineeringwatch.org

We were also reminded that we do live in Amarillo, Texas, the home of Pantex. I was born and raised in Amarillo and so was Courtney. Pantex is the primary United States nuclear weapons assembly and disassembly facility that aims to maintain the safety, security, and reliability of the U.S. nuclear weapons stockpile. The facility is located on a 16,000-acre site 17 miles northeast of Amarillo, in Carson County, Texas in the Panhandle of Texas.

The Gardasil and flu vaccines are what almost caused Courtney's death in 2015. Do you remember her home saliva hormone test? Remember it showed that she was premenopausal? The Gardasil vaccine caused that!

She has all detox pathways open and her body has detoxed, thank you Plexus! And her brain has detoxed, thank you Dr. Pompa! I have my social butterfly back!

January 5, 2019, after her chiropractic treatment we took advantage of the beautiful weather and went for a walk. We walked around our local elementary school not once, but twice! Courtney was going so fast I had a hard time keeping up with her! The OCD symptoms she had been experiencing were decreasing and the social anxiety was lifting! Thank God!!!

January 18, 2019, her chiropractor, Dr. Jack Mustard, said she was getting healthy! A lot of people had been saying this! So good to hear. Praise God! God led us to the right people and the right tools. Thanksgiving Day 2018 she was in a wheelchair after getting an amalgam (silver) filling removed October 2018. Dr. Jack Mustard helped her to walk again! Thank you, Dr. Mustard! She had been playing with her dog Little Bit again too! The last time I saw her playing with him was when he was a puppy, he was 3 years old at this point. She could not play with him because of the OCD that plagued her because she was afraid of his "germs" and him getting her dirty.

February 1, 2019, Courtney's grandmama, Courtney and I went for a walk twice around our closest elementary school. I ate Courtney's dust. I kept thinking, Thanksgiving Day 2018 she was in a wheelchair. I praise God every day for leading us to Plexus supplements, Young Living essential oils, our K8 Kangen water system, Mrs. Jane Remington (author of *Recaging the Beast*), Dr. Jack Mustard, Robert Sherry (a friend who had personal experience with Dr. Pompa's supplements) and Dr. Daniel Pompa.

Courtney never saw Dr. Daniel Pompa as a client, she was only taking his Cytodetox, Bind and brain phase. Robert Sherry was kind enough to coach Courtney since I could not afford Dr. Daniel Pompa's coaching.

April 26, 2019, we had been able to add raw zucchini, blueberries, red potatoes and pears to Courtney's diet!

June 14, 2019, Courtney continued to amaze me! It was amazing that she was in a wheelchair Thanksgiving Day of 2018, only 6 months ago! Here she is shooting basketball hoops with her cousin Creed!

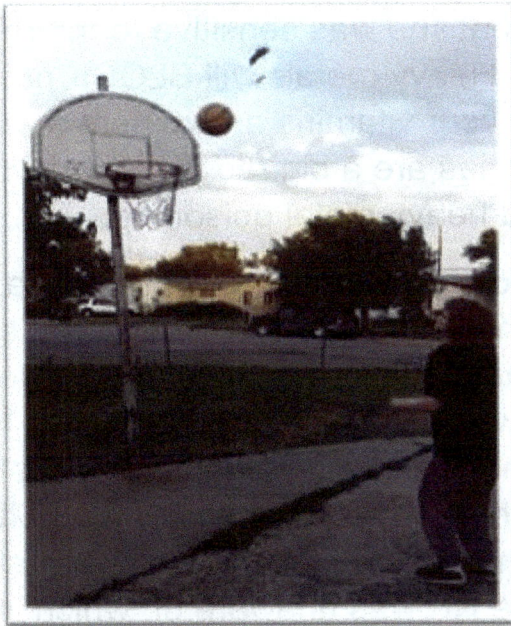

I am so thankful to God for showing me the way to Plexus supplements, Young Living essential oils, our K8 Kangen water system, nutrition and an excellent holistic chiropractor.

Before she started detoxing from the heavy metals, her stomach was having a hard time handling the red potatoes.

Her prior alternative NP was surprised that her stomach was having a hard time with the red potatoes since they are an ingredient in Hippocrates soup.

Therefore, we muscle tested her and it showed that she was sensitive to the red potatoes. Heavy metals will BLOCK nutrition and steal your vitamins and minerals. Multiple food allergies are a big red flag for vaccine injury and heavy metal poisoning.

Since following Dr. Daniel Pompa, I had learned that the reason for Courtney's seizure was because the heavy metal detox protocol that she was using with the alternative NP, was working against the amalgam filling. Before detoxing heavy metals specially, you MUST remove the source first. This was something her alternative NP was unaware of, which is the reason why Courtney has not been back to that NP. I still follow Dr. Daniel Pompa. Since getting her amalgam filling removed Courtney has not experienced another seizure.

November 5, 2019, Courtney was behind the wheel again! She was 27 years old!

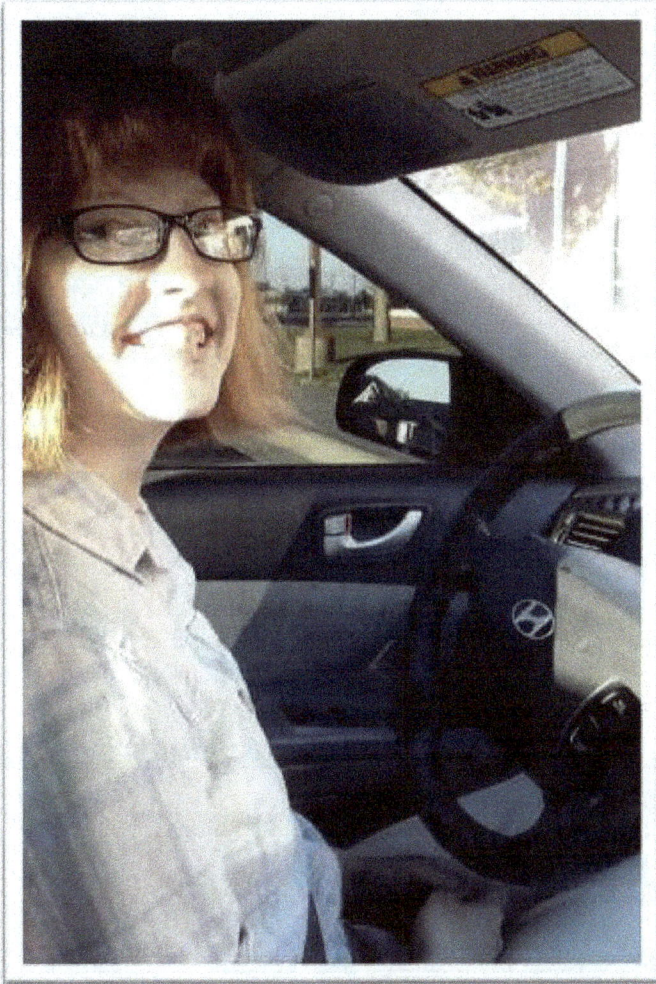

We are now ex-vaxxers and we do not take any medications!

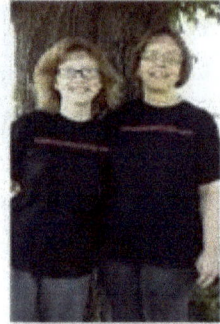

Candida Overgrowth,
Vaccine Injury &
Heavy Metals Poisoning
Healing Journey
www.CompassionWithKim.com

kim.seymore@sbcglobal.net

Follow us on Facebook, MeWe and Parler.
Watch us on YouTube.

https://www.facebook.com/kimdseymour

https://mewe.com/i/kimseymour3

https://mewe.com/i/courtneyseymour

https://parler.com/profile/KimSeymore/posts

https://parler.com/profile/Courtneyseymour1121/posts

https://www.youtube.com/channel/UCEge7k6MMmV8JHAGfp8pCiQ?view_as=subscriber